*Our "Compacted" Compact Clinicals Team*

# Dear Valued Customer,

**W**ELCOME to Compact Clinicals. We are committed to bringing mental health professionals up-to-date diagnostic and treatment information in a compact, timesaving, and easy-to-read format. Our line of books provides current, thorough reviews of assessment and treatment strategies for mental disorders.

We've "compacted" complete information for diagnosing each disorder and comparing how different theoretical orientations approach treatment. Our books use nonacademic language, real-world examples, and well-defined terminology.

Enjoy this and other timesaving books from Compact Clinicals.

Sincerely,

*Melanie A. Dean*

Melanie Dean, Ph.D.
President

# Compact Clinicals Line of Books

*Compact Clinicals currently offers these condensed reviews for professionals:*

## For Clinicians

### Attention Deficit Hyperactivity Disorder
*The latest assessment and treatment strategies*
> C. Keith Conners, Ph.D.

### Bipolar Disorder
*The latest assessment and treatment strategies*
> Trisha Suppes M.D., Ph.D., and Ellen B. Dennehy, Ph.D.

### Borderline Personality Disorder
*The latest assessment and treatment strategies*
> Melanie Dean, Ph.D.

### Conduct Disorders
*The latest assessment and treatment strategies*
> J. Mark Eddy, Ph.D.

### Depression in Adults
*The latest assessment and treatment strategies*
> Anton Tolman, Ph.D.

### Obsessive Compulsive Disorder
*The latest assessment and treatment strategies*
> Gail Steketee, Ph.D., and Teresa Pigott, M.D.

### Post-Traumatic and Acute Stress Disorders
*The latest assessment and treatment strategies*
> Matthew Friedman, M.D., Ph.D.

## For Physicians

### Bipolar Disorder: Treatment and Management
Trisha Suppes, M.D., Ph.D., and Paul E. Keck, Jr., M.D.

# Borderline Personality Disorder

*The latest assessment and treatment strategies*

### Third Edition

Melanie Dean, Ph.D.

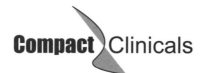

This book is intended for use by properly trained and licensed mental health professionals, who already possess a solid education in psychological theory, research, and treatment. This book is in no way intended to replace or supplement such training and education, nor is it to be used as the sole basis for any decision regarding treatment. It is merely intended to be used by such trained and educated professionals as a review and resource guide when considering how to best treat borderline personality disorder.

## Borderline Personality Disorder

*The latest assessment and treatment strategies*

Third Edition

by

Melanie Dean, Ph.D.

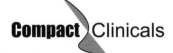

Published by: Compact Clinicals
7205 NW Waukomis Dr., Suite A
Kansas City, MO 64151
816-587-0044

©2006 Dean Psych Press Corp. d/b/a Compact Clinicals

**Medical Editing:** Kathi Whitman, In Credible English, Inc.,®
Kansas City, Missouri

**Book Design:** Coleridge Design, Kansas City, Missouri

**Library of Congress Cataloging in Publication data:**

Dean, Melanie A.
Borderline personality disorder : the latest assessment and treatment strategies / by Melanie A. Dean. — 3rd ed.
        p.    ;    cm.
    Includes bibliographical references and index.
    ISBN-13: 978-1-887537-20-9
    ISBN-10: 1-887537-20-1
    1. Borderline personality disorder—Handbooks, manuals, etc.
[DNLM: 1. Borderline Personality Disorder—diagnosis—Handbooks.
2. Borderline Personality Disorder—therapy—Handbooks. WM 34 D282b 2006]
I. Title.

  RC569.5.B67D43 2006
  616.85'852—dc22
            2005034241

10  9  8  7  6  5  4  3  2  1

# Read Me First

As a mental health professional, often the information you need can only be obtained after countless hours of reading or library research. If your schedule precludes this time commitment, Compact Clinicals is the answer.

Our books are practitioner oriented with easy-to-read treatment descriptions and examples. Compact Clinicals books are written in a nonacademic style. Our books are formatted to make the first reading, as well as ongoing reference, quick and easy. You will find:

► *Anecdotes* — Each chapter contains a fictionalized account that personalizes the disorder entitled, "From the Patient's Perspective."

► *Sidebars* — Narrow columns on the outside of each page highlight important information, preview upcoming sections or concepts, and define terms used in the text.

► *Definitions* — Terms are defined in the sidebars where they originally appear in the text and in an alphabetical glossary on pages 65 through 69.

► *References* — Numbered references appear in the text following information from that source. Full references appear on pages 71 through 79.

► *Case Examples* — Our examples illustrate typical adult client comments or conversational exchanges that help clarify different treatment approaches. Identifying information in the examples (e.g., the individual's real name, profession, age, and/or location) has been changed to protect the confidentiality of those clients discussed in case examples.

► *Key Concepts* — At the end of each chapter, we include a review list of key concepts from that chapter. Use these lists for ongoing quick reference as well as for reviewing what you learned from reading the chapter.

# Contents

# Chapter One:
## Overview of Borderline Personality Disorder

*This chapter answers the following:*

► **How Common is Borderline Personality Disorder (BPD)?** — This section discusses prevalence rates (recurrence) in terms of gender, age, and race.

► **What is the Likelihood of Recovery for those with BPD?** — This section discusses prognosis and includes both positive and negative predictors of recovery.

**M**ILLIONS of Americans suffer from borderline personality disorder (referred to throughout this book as "BPD"), a pervasive pattern of instability that begins early in life and affects most of a person's daily functioning.

People with BPD suffer from emotional and behavioral instability that begins at an early age and remains persistent throughout their lives. They primarily suffer from intense fears that significant others will leave them and react to these intense fears with manipulation, intense anger, and other volatile behaviors to preserve important relationships. In addition, people with BPD fear their need for others. This results in emotional extremes from anger to sadness to euphoria coupled with erratic and often dangerous behavior. They typically have one or more addictions (e.g., alcohol, spending money, gambling, drugs, or sex) and frequently respond to their unstable emotions through self mutilation (e.g., cutting on one's self), suicidal thoughts, or suicidal behavior.

BPD symptoms range from mild to very severe. Inpatient psychiatric hospitals often admit people diagnosed with BPD who have extreme symptoms, including suicidal and/or homicidal thoughts (or behaviors) or attempts. In an outpatient setting, those with this disorder are likely to have:

► Symptoms of depression

► Suicidal ideation

► Decreased functioning in one or more areas of their lives (e.g., unable to hold a job, marital strife)

The characterization of those with BPD has evolved over several decades with the first written work published in the 1930s. The original document described patients with BPD as occupying a continuum between *neurosis* and *psychosis*. The disorder remained vague through the 1940s, and those with BPD were tagged as "pseudoneurotic schizophrenic." The current definition has changed little and illustrates both the *maladaptive behavior patterns* and the mild psychotic symptoms often displayed by

*Written for the professional, this book presents general information about BPD in chapter one, diagnostic information in chapter two, various theoretical etiologies and psychotherapeutic treatments in chapter three, and medications in chapter four.*

**neurosis** — non-physiological disorder characterized by high levels of anxiety but no impairment in reality testing

**psychosis** — grossly impaired reality testing

**maladaptive behavior patterns** — patterns of behavior likely to produce so much psychic distress that therapy is necessary

1

people with BPD. Current research debates center around the origin of the disorder and whether BPD is better classified as part of the bipolar spectrum of mood disorders with prominent affective instability.[1-3] Research estimates indicate that at least 44 percent of those with BPD have prominent bipolar symptoms.[4]

Correctly identifying bipolar is important because antidepressant therapy, the most common BPD medication treatment, induces mood switches to mania or hypomania. The estimates of bipolarity in BPD are as high as 69 percent when antidepressant-induced hypomania is taken into consideration.[4]

## How Common is Borderline Personality Disorder (BPD)?

Calculations of community prevalence rates for BPD range from two to 6.5 percent.[5-7] Based on a U.S. population of approximately 250 million, these statistics indicate that five to 16 million people suffer from this disorder. A 1982 cross-cultural study indicated a 15 to 20 percent prevalence rate among psychiatric inpatients.[5] Prevalence rates for outpatient mental health clinics are about 10 percent.[8]

**Gender** — Women are diagnosed with BPD two to four times more often than men.[9, 10] These results may highlight real differences between men and women or result from a labeling difference. Men with similar symptoms are more often diagnosed as having either antisocial personality disorder (APD) or narcissistic personality disorder (NPD).

**Age** — The highest rates of diagnosed BPD are found in those between the ages of 19 and 34.[10]

**Race** — Differences between races in terms of diagnoses suggest that other races are diagnosed as BPD at a significantly higher rate than Caucasians.[10]

## From The Patient's Perspective

*We had another fight last night. Alex just doesn't understand. Says I'm drinking too much. I feel so alone; nobody is ever there for me. I just feel like cutting on myself again. I hate this, seems like people have been leaving me all my life. I hope Alex doesn't find out I didn't come home last night. Started seeing a therapist named Pat Owen. She's going to be great. Owen says I may have BPD but says there are a lot of ways to get better.*

# What is the Likelihood of Recovery for those with BPD?

The few studies conducted assessing treatment effectiveness indicate a poor, short-term prognosis for those diagnosed with BPD. These studies found that subjects had chronic symptoms, high relapse rates, and poor employment as well as significant impairment at work and in relationships with others.[11-13] Some research indicates that about 50 percent of those with BPD tend to stabilize, contending with fewer BPD symptoms over time.[14] Specifically, dysphoria, impulsiveness, disturbed relationships, and *micropsychotic symptoms* tend to decrease over time, with about 75 percent of patients no longer meeting full criteria for BPD by age 40.[15-18] However, other research suggests that patients experience persistent symptoms and adapt to their changing needs with age.[19]

**micropsychotic symptoms** — minor psychotic symptoms

Completed suicides during the most dysfunctional periods of the disorder range from three to 10 percent with most studies indicating nine percent.[15, 20, 21] This is quite high when compared to the .00011 percent suicide rate among the general U.S. population.[22]

*Pages 16 and 52 through 55 feature information on dealing with suicide risk.*

Figure 1.1, below, lists factors associated with completed suicides for those suffering from BPD. These factors indicate that patients with less severe BPD symptomatology and traumatic history have higher suicide rates. They were more functional in reality testing, more able to form relationships, and more hopeful about the future (as a result of more education). This higher level of functioning may make the emotional struggles related to BPD seem intolerable. Lower functioning people with BPD, who experienced more trauma and difficulty early in life, may have adapted and thus have a higher level of tolerance.

*Figure 1.2, on the next page, illustrates indicators of positive and negative suicide outcomes.*

**Figure 1.1   Factors Associated with Completed Suicides in People with BPD[15]**

- ▶ Presence of depression.[23]
- ▶ Mean age of those completing suicide is 32.9.
- ▶ Mean time of suicide is four years after inpatient hospitalization.
- ▶ Those who successfully complete suicide generally:
  - ▷ Attempted suicide in the past
  - ▷ Were more highly educated than survivors
  - ▷ Had fewer psychotic symptoms than survivors
  - ▷ Reported fewer problems with their mothers than survivors
  - ▷ Suffered fewer separations and losses before the age of five
- ▶ No difference exists between people who complete suicide and survivors in terms of age, sex, marital status, conflict with fathers, and substance abuse.

### Figure 1.2    Suicide Prognosis Predictors

| Predictors of positive prognosis include:[14, 24, 25] | Predictors of negative prognosis include:[24-27] |
|---|---|
| • Shorter hospitalizations* <br> • Presence of distractibility <br> • Presence of self-destructive acts during hospitalizations (not self-destructive acts prior to hospitalization) <br> • Absence of: <br>   – Affective instability <br>   – Parental divorce <br>   – Feelings of entitlement <br>   – Feelings of boredom <br>   – Impulsivity | • History of childhood sexual abuse <br> • Substance abuse <br> • Prominent antisocial traits <br> • Dysphoria (mild chronic depression) <br> • Multiple mental disorders |

\* The presence of self-destructive acts during hospitalization is a positive (even if surprising) predictor. This behavior may reflect a readiness to receive help and destructive acting out in such a setting allows patients to learn alternate coping skills.

## Key Concepts for Chapter One:

1. Borderline personality disorder (BPD) is a pervasive pattern of emotional and behavioral instability that affects much of a person's daily functioning.

2. Characteristic symptoms of BPD range from depression and decreased functioning in one or more areas of life to suicidal or homicidal thoughts and behaviors.

3. BPD appears to be most prevalent among those aged 19 to 34, among women, and among those of races other than Caucasian.

4. Although many patients with BPD can achieve stability over time with treatment, risk of suicide during dysfunctional periods is high.

# Chapter Two:
## Diagnosing and Assessing
## Borderline Personality Disorder

### This chapter answers the following:

▶ **What Criteria Are Used to Diagnose BPD?** — This section reviews DSM-IV (TR) diagnostic criteria for BPD.

▶ **What are Typical Characteristics of Those with BPD?** — This section covers clinical presentation as well as subgroups of BPD.

▶ **What Tools are Used for Clinical Assessment?** — This section covers clinical assessment methods, including interview questions, self-report measures, and psychometric assessment tools.

▶ **How is BPD Differentiated from Other Disorders?** — This section helps differentiate BPD from other personality and affective disorders that may present similar symptoms.

## What Criteria Are Used to Diagnose BPD?

THE *Diagnostic and Statistical Manual of Mental Disorders-Fourth Edition, Text Revision [DSM-IV(TR)]* provides the most current criteria for diagnosing BPD (see figure 2.2 on the next page).[8] Much debate exists over the subjectiveness of each criterion. Clinicians should be aware that these criteria define a nonspecific type of serious character pathology rather than a specific, well-defined disorder.[28]

> Diagnosis of BPD must reflect observation of ongoing patterns of behavior rather than one-time reactions to specific events. Behaviors must lead to functional impairment in the vocational and/or social areas of the person's life.

### Diagnostic Research

The DSM-IV (TR) criteria appear to cluster around three primary factors that are statistically significant: disturbed relationships, behavioral dysregulation, and effective dysregulation.[29] Depending on the setting, various indicators appear to be best for diagnosing BPD (see figure 2.1). Of all the diagnostic criteria, stress-related paranoia is the least predictive of BPD.[30]

### Figure 2.1 Best BPD Diagnostic Indicators

| Inpatient[30, 31] | Outpatient[32] |
|---|---|
| • Abandonment | • Unstable/intense relationships |
| • Unstable relationships | • Chronic boredom |
| • Impulsivity | • Feelings of emptiness |
| • Physically self-damaging acts | |

## Figure 2.2   DSM-IV(TR) Criteria for BPD

"A pervasive pattern of instability of interpersonal relationships, self-image and affects, and marked impulsivity beginning by early adulthood and present in a variety of contexts, as indicated by five or more of the following:

1. frantic efforts to avoid real or imagined abandonment
   **Note: Do not include suicidal or self-mutilating behavior covered in Criterion 5.**

2. a pattern of unstable and intense interpersonal relationships characterized by alternating between extremes of *idealization* and *devaluation*

3. identity disturbance: markedly and persistently unstable self-image or sense of self

4. impulsivity in at least two areas that are potentially self-damaging (e.g., spending, sex, substance abuse, reckless driving, binge eating)
   **Note: Do not include suicidal or self-mutilating behavior covered in Criterion 5.**

5. recurrent suicidal behavior, gestures, or threats, or self-mutilation behavior

6. affective instability due to a marked reactivity of mood (e.g., intense episodic dysphoria, irritability, or anxiety usually lasting a few hours and only rarely more than a few days)

7. chronic feelings of emptiness

8. inappropriate, intense anger or difficulty controlling anger (e.g., frequent displays of temper, constant anger, recurrent physical fights)

9. transient, stress-related paranoid ideation or severe dissociative symptoms."

Reprinted with permission of American Psychiatric Association, *Diagnostic Statistical Manual of Mental Disorders, Fourth Edition (Text Revision)*, Washington D.C., American Psychiatric Association, 2000.[8]

**idealization** — the process whereby the patient sees another person as only "good" or "perfect"

**devaluation** — the process whereby the patient under-values the abilities and/or intentions of others

*Diagnostic Note: Many terms or phrases used in DSM-IV(TR) criteria highlight the importance of historical information in diagnosing BPD (e.g.,"pervasive," "chronic," "persistent," "frequent," and "pattern of"). Not only must current behavior fit the criteria, historical information must support a long-term pattern of such behavior. If current behavior fits the diagnosis while past behavior does not, then alternate diagnoses need to be considered (e.g., adjustment disorder, affective disorder, or psychotic disorder).*

When researching patients' past behavioral history, researchers discovered the following commonalities among those with moderate-to-severe BPD:[33]

▶ Frequent suicide attempts

▶ Inpatient discharges against medical advice

▶ First suicide attempt before age 40

▶ Violence within and outside the hospital

▶ Gradual deterioration in social/occupational functioning

Often those with BPD suffer from chronic diseases, such as fibromyalgia, chronic fatigue, obesity, diabetes, osteoarthritis, back pain, or urinary incontinence, and utilize medications and health services to a significantly greater extent than patients whose BPD is in "remission."[34]

# What are Typical Characteristics of Those with BPD?

During the initial assessment interview and in subsequent treatment sessions, the clinician can recognize patients with BPD through several common features: [35, 36]

1. **Disturbance in Self Concept** — People with BPD typically have a highly variable self-image. They generally base their self-image on what others say about them or reactions they receive from others. For example, someone with BPD who receives a critical comment from a coworker may decide, "I am a terrible person." After a compliment, the same person will think, "I am wonderful and perfect." This variability in self-image leads to wide mood swings and contradictory thoughts about oneself.

   The variability in self-image is often emotionally painful due to the distress of interpreting experiences negatively and personally. In addition, the identity disturbance is associated with a lack of commitment due to values, occupations, and relationships fluctuating rapidly along with changes in the person's self-view.[37]

2. **Unstable Interpersonal Relationships** — People with BPD have a strong need for dependable relationships and are also overly sensitive to others' emotions.[38] This sensitivity and dependence on others often results in using indirect and subtle methods for gaining support, such as over-idealizing or devaluing the perceived supporter. Those closest to someone with BPD often perceive this behavior as "manipulative" and fail to see the person's underlying needs. Typically, the person with BPD does not consciously admit a need for others and pushes them away during times of stress. This push-and-pull behavior often leads to short-lived relationships with intense beginnings and endings.

3. **Cognitive Disturbances** — When dealing with severe stress, people with BPD may suffer from transient psychotic symptoms including *dissociation*, *derealization*, *depersonalization*, and *paranoia*. Individuals that are at particular risk for cognitive disturbances are those who suffered inconsistent treatment or sexual abuse by a caretaker, witnessed sexual violence as a child, or were adult victims of rape.[40]

4. **Impulsive Behaviors** — *Impulsive* behaviors about eating, shopping, and gambling often occur with BPD. The most prevalent impulsive (and *compulsive*) behavior

*Common Features of People with BPD*

1. Disturbance in Self Concept
2. Unstable Interpersonal Relationships
3. Cognitive Disturbances
4. Impulsive Behaviors
5. Labile Affect
6. Functional Failures
7. Self-Destructive Acts

*Those with BPD fear separation from others and cannot tolerate feelings of being alone.[20] Sometimes this condition is described as "abandonment depression" leading those with BPD to be socially overactive and compulsive to avoid being alone.[39]*

**dissociation** — an abnormal psychological state in which one's perception of oneself and/or one's environment is altered significantly

**derealization** — a sense that one has lost contact with external reality

*continued*

*continued*

**depersonalization** — a sense that one has lost contact with one's own personal reality (e.g., "My body feels strange, like it's not my own.")

**paranoia** — having suspicions and beliefs that one is being followed, plotted against, persecuted, etc.

**impulsive** — acting without first thinking about the action

**compulsive** — feeling compelled to act against one's wishes

**labile affect** — marked and rapid mood shifts

**affect** — emotion; feeling; mood

*Page 3 summarizes risk factors for suicidal behavior with more detail covered on page 16 in chapter two. Additionally, pages 52 through 55 review treatment issues key to helping suicidal patients.*

involves alcohol and other drug abuse, especially among young adults.[14, 35] Another common impulsive and often addictive behavior is sexual promiscuity or deviance.

5. *Labile Affect* — People with BPD have sudden, frequent, and intense changes in *affect*.[14, 35] Anger, emptiness, loneliness, or abandonment may be expressed as rage or as bitterness and despondency. During times of intense affect, the demands on others for attention and support will likely increase.

   Research indicates that those with BPD experience both higher levels of unpleasant emotions and greater fluctuations in pleasant emotions.[41, 42] Specifically, there are often higher rates of anger, hostility and aggressive affects in those with BPD.[43] This labile affect appears to be related to a difficulty in recognizing and regulating emotion. Those with BPD often have lower levels of emotional awareness and less ability to accurately identify emotional facial expressions of others. Additionally, they have less capacity to manage mixed emotions and tend to over respond in intensity to the negative emotions of others.[7, 44]

   In summary, research indicates that difficulty in regulating emotion is a hallmark dysfunction for those with BPD.

6. **Functional Failures** — Many people with BPD are unable to successfully apply their abilities. They show potential for high achievement; however, their emotional instability and cognitive disturbances prevent them from reaching that potential.

7. **Self-Destructive Activity** — The most extreme self-destructive behavior is suicide (nearly 10 percent of those with BPD complete suicide).[11, 45, 46] Other self-harm activities include cutting on the body, ingestion of harmful substances, and genital mutilation. Often those with BPD dissociate during self-mutilation and following mutilation feel happier and less dissociative.[47] Alcohol and drug abuse are frequent problems for those with BPD.[48] Additionally, self-destructive behavior overlaps with impulsive behavior on occasion. For example, eating disorders are common among people with BPD.

## Subgroups of BPD

People diagnosed with BPD may appear very different from each other. These variations reflect three primary subgroups (see figure 2.3 below) of patients who:

1. Are primarily depressed
2. Are primarily impulsive
3. Present symptoms that are primarily psychotic

These subgroups are not mutually exclusive; clients can manifest symptoms from one or all of the subgroups. The chart below (figure 2.3) presents the symptoms and related disorders for each subgroup.

### Figure 2.3   BPD Subgroups

| | Symptoms | Related Disorders* |
|---|---|---|
| **Primarily: Depressed** | • Chronic depression<br>• A demanding, dramatic interpersonal style<br>• Atypical depressive symptoms of reactivity, lability, rejection-sensitivity, *hyperphrasia*, and hypersomnia | • Major depression, atypical depression, and dysthymia |
| **Primarily: Impulsive** | • Overdose<br>• Suicide threats<br>• Self-mutilation<br>• Alcohol or other drug binges<br>• Sexual promiscuity<br>• Antisocial acts | • Bipolar affective disorder<br>• Cyclothymia<br>• Antisocial personality disorder (APD)<br>• Organic disorders (including post-traumatic stress disorder, seizure-associated and attention deficit hyperactivity disorder) |
| **Primarily: Psychotic\*\*** | • Paranoia<br>• *Referential thinking*<br>• Depersonalization, derealization<br>• *Delusions*<br>• *Hallucinations*<br>• Odd experiences<br>• *Mild formal thought disorder* | • Schizotypal personality disorder (SPD)<br>• Brief reactive psychosis<br>• Atypical psychosis |

\* These represent disorders with which there is a high dual diagnosis and/or correlation of symptoms with BPD.

\*\* Multiple stress-related, psychotic-like symptoms are usually transient. Psychotic-like symptoms are most often mood congruent (e.g., paranoid ideation or referential thinking patients would have depressive and poor self- image content congruent with their depressive mood.) Brief, supportive hospitalizations are often sufficient to control these symptoms.

**hyperphrasia** — pathologically excessive talking

**referential thinking** — mistakenly believing others' actions or external events are specifically related to one's self

**delusions** — beliefs maintained despite much evidence or argument to the contrary

**hallucinations** — hearing or seeing things others do not

**mild formal thought disorder** — disturbances in speech, communication, and/or thinking

# What Tools are Used for Clinical Assessment?

Several tools can help the clinician diagnose BPD, including the clinical interview, self-report and interview instruments, and psychometric assessment tools.

## Clinical Interview

During the initial interview, the clinician needs to specifically ask about certain factors that can help diagnose BPD, such as:

> ▶ Historical patterns of substance abuse, gambling, money-spending binges, or promiscuity (indications of impulsive symptoms)

> ▶ Intense beginnings and endings of relationships and cutoff relationships with family members (indicators of unstable relationships)

> ▶ Psychotic-like symptoms, such as depersonalization, derealization, delusions, hallucinations, paranoia, and referential thinking

> ▶ History of sexual, physical or emotional abuse

> ▶ Suicide attempts, self-mutilation, binging and purging, or not eating (indicators of self-destructive behavior)

*Many people with BPD have experienced significant trauma.*

### Talking with Patients about Suicide

It is critical in the clinical interview to determine whether or not the patient may be a suicide risk. Ask clear, simple questions about whether or not the patient wants to die and if they have a plan for committing suicide. The goal is to determine how emotionally upset or unstable the person is, how likely the person is to act on their suicidal ideation, and how difficult it would be to rescue the person if they were to use the method they are considering. Utilize an "ascending approach" for the patient interview, beginning with questions about nonspecific suicidal thinking, then moving into a review of specific passive and active suicidal thoughts.[49] Nonspecific suicidal thinking involves questions like:

> ▶ "Have you ever thought of hurting yourself?"

> ▶ "Have you had suicidal thoughts recently?"

Reviewing specific passive suicidal thoughts might involve asking questions like:

> ▶ "Do you want to commit suicide?"

> ▶ "Might you do so sometime if things get worse?"

- ▶ "Do you think about suicide but have no specific plans?"
- ▶ "Do you sometimes wish you could die?"

Reviewing specific active suicidal thoughts might involve asking:

- ▶ "When are you planning to commit suicide?"
- ▶ "How would you do that? What method are you planning to use?"
- ▶ "Where do you think about killing yourself?"

The clinician then asks for a description of all methods the patient has used in the past and evaluates how much time and effort the patient has expended in considering current suicide plans. This information is vital because the patient is likely to repeat past behaviors. Certain methods of attempting suicide are much more lethal or dangerous than others; for example, attempting suicide by shooting oneself is much more likely to result in death than attempting an overdose.

*Patients who have made use of more lethal methods in the past tend to be more:*

- ▶ *Serious about actually dying*
- ▶ *Disappointed that they did not succeed with previous attempts*
- ▶ *Likely to use highly lethal methods in future attempts*

Similarly, if a person has a history of prior attempts, it is very important to understand why they did not die. For example, if the person wakes up and calls for help, it indicates some desire to live. On the other hand, if the only reason the person did not die was that they pulled the gun's trigger too hard and the bullet did not strike a critical area, such a patient should be considered a much higher risk.

The presence of multiple attempts, especially of low lethality, is likely to indicate the presence of a personality disorder, as compared with an acute clinical disorder. Capturing a solid clinical history of prior attempts is directly relevant to developing an effective treatment plan for reducing depression and the risk for future suicide.

## From The Patient's Perspective

*Saw my therapist, Pat Owen, today. She's perfect. This time I'm going to get fixed. She wants me to take some tests. Already I feel better. I haven't thought about suicide in days or cutting on myself. Work is bad, though; everybody is out to get me fired.*

*Got back together with Alex; I just know this will last forever.*

## Self-Report and Interview Instruments

**Self-report instruments** available to assess and diagnose BPD include:

▶ **Borderline Personality Inventory** — This instrument is based on a psychodynamic formulation of BPD, while also compatible with DSM-IV (TR) diagnostic criteria. It assesses four areas:

  ▶ Identity diffusion

  ▶ Primitive defense mechanisms

  ▶ Reality testing

  ▶ Fear of closeness

In addition to the descriptive validity scales, a cutoff score can be used to diagnose BPD. The instrument shows good reliability, *sensitivity*, and *specificity* data for diagnosis.[50]

**sensitivity ratio** — cases correctly diagnosed

**specificity ratio** — non-cases correctly identified

▶ **McLean Screening Instrument for Borderline Personality Disorder (MSI-BPD)** — This 10-item screening tool for BPD has good sensitivity (.81 correctly identified cases) as well as specificity (.85 correctly identified non-cases) based on DSM-IV (TR) diagnostic criteria for BPD.[51] For younger subjects, sensitivity was .90 and specificity was .93.

▶ **Objective Behavioral Index** — This index assesses treatment response in clients with severe personality disorders. It measures dysfunctional behaviors as well as use of mental health services.[52]

▶ **Personality Assessment Inventory (PAI)** — This 344-item inventory has 22 scales, including validity, clinical, treatment, and interpersonal scales with four borderline feature subscales: Affective Instability, Identity Problems, Negative Relationships, and Self-Harm. This instrument has good reliability and *validity* data and can also be used for diagnosing BPD.[53-55]

**validity** — degree that the instrument measures what it purports to measure

**Interview instruments** available to assess and diagnose BPD include:

▶ **Diagnostic Interview for Borderline Personality Disorders-Revised (DIB-R)**[56] — Based on DSM criteria, this instrument has strong sensitivity and specificity for diagnosis. The DIB-R reliably distinguishes BPD from other Axis II personality disorders. It consists of a one-hour, semi-structured interview focusing on social adaptation, self-destructive impulsiveness, depressive and angry affect, *dissociative ego states*, and interpersonal relations.

**dissociative ego states** — attitudes and emotions that produce anxiety become separated from the rest of the person's personality and function independently

▶ **Structured Clinical Interview for DSM-III-R Personality Disorders (SCID-II)**[57] — Designed as a guide for diagnostic interviewing using DSM-III-R criteria, the SCID-II contains sections for both Axis I and II disorders. The Axis II portion of the interview includes diagnostic questions for 11 different DSM-III-R personality disorders. This instrument demonstrates strong sensitivity, specificity, validity, and *inter-rater reliability*.[58-59]

▶ **Zanarini Rating Scale for Borderline Personality Disorder (ZAN-BPD)** — This clinician-administered scale is the first developed to assess change in DSM-IV borderline psychopathology. It was adapted from the BPD module of the Diagnostic Interview for DSM-IV Personality Disorders (DIPD-IV), reflecting a one-week time frame with each criterion rated on a five-point scale. In a study of the ZAN-BPD's psychometric properties, the tool showed highly significant *convergent validity*, *discriminant validity*, and inter-rater reliability, making it a highly promising tool for measuring change in a clinically significant manner.[60]

**inter-rater reliability** — degree that different raters agree on a diagnosis based on the use of the instrument

**convergent validity** — when test results positively correlate with other instruments measuring the same variable

**discriminant validity** — an instrument's ability to discriminate BPD from other disorders

*See page 16 for a discussion on assessing suicide risk.*

Instruments for assessing suicide and self-harm include:

▶ **Self-Harm Inventory (SHI)** — This instrument identifies self-destructive behaviors and is useful as a screening tool for BPD. It is a 22-item, semi-structured inventory showing preliminary validity for diagnosis.[61]

▶ **Beck Scale for Suicide Ideation** — This scale is a self-administered, 21-item scale assessing frequency and content of suicidal ideation for clinician follow-up.[62]

▶ **Suicide Probability Scale (SPS)** — This is a 36-item, self-administered scale offering a suicide probability score and detailed information on four subscales: Hopelessness, Suicide Ideation, Negative Self Evaluation, and Hostility.[63]

## Psychometric Assessment Tools

Psychometric instruments that are commonly used for diagnosis also include:

▶ Minnesota Multiphasic Personality Inventory (MMPI)

▶ Wechsler Adult Intelligence Scale-Revised (WAIS-R)

▶ Rorschach

▶ Millon Clinical Multi-Axial Inventory-II (MCMI)

**MMPI Scales**

L: Lie Scale

F: Fake Bad

K: Clinical Defensiveness

1: Hypochondriasis

2: Depression

3: Hysteria

4: Psychopathic Deviate

5: Masculinity/Femininity

6: Paranoia

7: Psychasthenia

8: Schizophrenia

9: Hypomania

10: Social Introversion

**Minnesota Multiphasic Personality Inventory-Second Edition (MMPI-2)** — The MMPI-2 is a widely used instrument assessing personality and symptoms of distress.[64] This test consists of 567 statements that the patient rates as either true or false. Clinicians score the test, often electronically, and construct a profile based on several specific scales.

Research findings suggest that those with BPD score high on both the "neurotic" (scales 1–4) and the "psychotic" (scales 6–8) MMPI scales. There is no clear pattern of MMPI-2 results that distinguishes BPD from other disorders. Commonalities among BPD profiles include an elevated F scale and an overall elevated profile (or "floating profile").[65] Typically, high scales are those numbered 2, 4, and 6 through 8.[53, 65] Some research indicates that scales F and 8 are almost always elevated and that scales L and K are typically less than 50.[66]

There are numerous books available to help interpret MMPI test results; the most frequently used are ones by Graham and Greene.[9, 67]

**Wechsler Adult Intelligence Scale (WAIS-R)** — The WAIS-R, like many other intelligence tests, was developed to:[68]

▶ Measure the patient's intellectual potential

▶ Obtain clinically relevant information pertaining to the patient's decision-making capacity

▶ Determine the ability to process language

▶ Assess the functional integrity of the brain

Rappaport's 1945 study led many to believe that those with BPD perform well on structured tests, such as the WAIS-R. The same study indicated that these people performed poorly, often with signs of thought disorder, on unstructured projective tests.[69] Subsequent studies do not support this research.[66] Typical WAIS-R results for BPD clients show few instances of thought disorder, relatively intact picture completion, and easy errors on comprehension questions. People with BPD show a wide range of WAIS-R profiles.[66]

**Rorschach** — This test is a *"projective" measure of personality*. It consists of 10 cards with randomly created inkblots, some in monochrome and some in color. The clinician shows the cards to the client one at a time, records the answers, and later scores them.

Although many systems score and interpret responses to the Rorschach test, the most widely used is the Exner Method, a comprehensive system for administering, scoring, and interpreting Rorschach results.[70]

**projective measure of personality (as measured by the Rorschach)** — the stimuli or inkblots are assumed to be neutral, created randomly with no specific shape nor function; patient perceptions of shapes, movement, and other elements seen as products of their own experiences and perceptual orientation projected on the cards

This is probably the best system to use for two reasons:

1. The Exner Method's large normative base allows the clinician to determine the irregularity of a particular score.

2. This system has survived extensive research on its validity and utility.

No simple profile has been identified for Rorschach findings when used to diagnose BPD. However, scores for those with BPD seem to show:[65, 66]

> Poorer capacity for behavior control (indicated by lower D scores).

> More involvement with the self at the expense of in-depth involvement with others (indicated by a higher egocentricity index).

> Evidence of minimum to moderate thought disorder with little to no evidence of severe thought disorder [demonstrated by few if any CONTAM (contamination), ALOG (autistic logic) and FABCOM (fabulized combination) scores]. High CONTAM scores successfully distinguish schizophrenics from those with BPD because that score almost exclusively predicts schizophrenia.

> Emotional overload or withdrawal (demonstrated by higher affective ratios).

> Poor perceptual accuracy (indicated by approximately 69 percent good form quality).

> Impaired capacity to regulate emotional arousal (demonstrated by high sum of shading and color responses).

**Millon Clinical Multi-Axial Inventory-II (MCMI-II)** — This self-report questionnaire assesses personality disorders for inpatients and is based on Millon's *taxonomy* for personality disorders.[71] However, the inventory provides inadequate convergent or discriminant validity for DSM Axis II personality disorders. MCMI-II fails to effectively diagnose BPD because Millon's theoretical orientation to personality disorders does not parallel DSM criteria.

*The information presented on Rorschach scores is intended for professionals trained in interpreting Rorschach results.*

**taxonomy** — classification system

**Predisposing Factors to Greater Suicide Risk**[23, 72–74]

▶ Being depressed

▶ Feeling hopeless

▶ Having an increase in impulsive aggression

▶ Living alone

▶ Being unmarried

▶ Being unemployed

▶ Having experienced recent loss

▶ Presenting a history of early parental loss

▶ History of childhood abuse

▶ Having a family history of suicide

▶ Having been recently discharged from hospitalization

▶ Having a severe physical illness

▶ Having a recent social failure

See pages 52 through 55 for a discussion on how to respond to suicide potential in patients with BPD.

**psychotropic medications** — medications that affect behavior, emotions, and/or cognitive processes

**electroconvulsive therapy (ECT)** — a type of treatment that induces a seizure through an external electrical source often used to treat depression

**psychotic depression** — severe depression that includes delusions (false beliefs) or hallucinations (perceptual distortions)

## Suicide Assessment

It is very difficult to accurately predict completed suicide. Thus, clinicians should focus on selecting the best strategy to effectively manage or lower suicide risk by reviewing predisposing factors and assessing whether or not the risk requires hospitalization). Key factors associated with suicide risk include:[75]

▶ **Previous suicide attempts that have been lethal in nature** — An indication of greater suicidal risk might be a serious overdose attempt (rather than ingestion of a dozen aspirin), or deep cutting on the wrists (versus superficial scratches).

▶ **The specificity of the suicide plan** — A patient that has worked out the time, circumstances, and means of committing suicide is more at risk than the patient who has no plan but admits to thinking about suicide.

▶ **The level of commitment to suicide and the availability of instruments** — A client who reports a "decision" to commit suicide is at greater risk than a client who reports "thinking" about suicide. In addition, someone who wants to overdose and has pills at home is more at risk than the person without a chosen suicide method readily available.

▶ **The level of impulsivity** — A client who generally exhibits impulsive behaviors in areas such as gambling, spending money, or beginning and ending relationships, is at greater risk for acting on their suicidal thoughts. The greater the impulsivity, the greater the suicide risk.[73]

▶ **The level of substance use** — The use of substances, particularly alcohol, leads to disinhibition and therefore greater risk for suicide, particularly with unplanned suicide attempts.[76]

▶ **The level of social support available** — People who have supportive friends and family to rely on are less likely to act on suicidal ideation.

Once the suicide risk level has been determined, the clinician can develop treatment strategies based on inpatient/outpatient considerations, the patient's history as a non- or single-attempter vs. a multiple-attempter, and what treatments are warranted.

Chapter three addresses psychological treatment strategies for suicidal patients. Biological treatments can include *psychotropic medications* or *electroconvulsive therapy (ECT)*. **Medications may be inappropriate for patients at imminent risk because they take a number of days to have an effect.** For patients who express suicide ideation and also refuse to eat, suffer from *psychotic depression*, or are at high risk for suicide and have not responded well to other treatments, ECT may be an appropriate alternative.

# How is BPD Differentiated from Other Disorders?

The BPD diagnostic category overlaps with other personality disorders, especially affective disorders; narcissistic, antisocial, histrionic, and schizotypal personality disorders; and post-traumatic stress disorder.[9] The table below (figure 2.4) differentiates each of these disorders from BPD.

## Figure 2.4 Differentiating BPD from Other Disorders

| Disorder | BPD Differential Diagnosis Guidelines |
|---|---|
| Antisocial Personality Disorder (APD) | • Those with BPD may perform antisocial acts, but are more likely to feel personal shame or remorse than those with APD.<br>• People with APD usually regret their actions only because of the consequences to themselves, not others.<br>• Antisocial acts committed by people with BPD are usually viewed as survival issues, and the individual experiences uncomfortable anxiety as a result. Those with APD usually feel no anxiety about their antisocial behavior. |
| Histrionic Personality Disorder (HPD) | • Those with HPD have a higher overall functional level, display greater employment and relationship stability, and maintain a more stable self-image.<br>• Those with HPD do not commit the repeated self-destructive acts typical of BPD.[11] |
| Narcissistic Personality Disorder (NPD) | • Those with BPD openly express their need for support in interpersonal relationships while those who are narcissistic are more subtle.<br>• Those with NPD typically deny their many dependency needs and are better able to have consistent and sustained relationships. People with BPD have more extreme affective displays and less stable relationships.<br>• NPD patients demonstrate grandiosity in contrast to the devalued sense of self evident in people with BPD.[6] |
| Schizotypal Personality Disorder (SPD) | • The flat affect that often accompanies BPD with depression is usually temporary or state-like (it lifts as the depression lifts). With SPD, flat affect is stable or trait-like.<br>• Clinicians view the psychotic symptoms present in those with SPD to be more trait-like, while similar symptoms among those with BPD are more transient, stress-related, or state-like.[77]<br>• Those with BPD have significantly higher rates of depression as well as substance abuse compared to those with SPD.[77] |
| Affective Disturbance (Depression, Dysthymia, Bipolar Disorder) | • Some researchers argue that BPD is a part of the affective disturbance spectrum. Others highlight the overlap between BPD and affective disturbance.[11]<br>• People who have affective instability, but who function well with minimal support and intervention, likely suffer from an affective disorder and would not meet BPD criteria. |
| Post-Traumatic Stress Disorder (PTSD) | • Those with BPD have often experienced significant trauma; however, they do not as a matter of course, experience PTSD symptoms (e.g., hypervigilance, exaggerated startle response, flashbacks, intrusive recollections, or efforts to avoid trauma-related thoughts and feelings).<br>• The dissociative symptoms associated with PTSD are a direct result of trauma-related stimuli rather than general stress-related dissociative symptoms seen with BPD.<br>• Many people with BPD also suffer from PTSD. |

## Key Concepts for Chapter Two

1. For inpatients, the best indicators of BPD include perceived abandonment, unstable relationships, impulsivity, and physically self-damaging acts.

2. Among outpatients, key BPD indicators include unstable and/or intense relationships, chronic boredom, and feelings of emptiness.

3. Those with moderate-to-severe BPD tend to have a history of frequent suicide attempts (first attempt before age 40), discharges from hospitals against medical advice, violence, and a gradual deterioration in social/occupational functioning.

4. Typical characteristics of BPD include disturbance in self concept, unstable relationships, cognitive disturbances, impulsivity, labile affect, functional failures, and self-destructive activity.

5. Key to interviewing a patient who has previously attempted suicide is to determine the lethality of the attempts, which can indicate presence of a personality disorder rather than an acute clinical disorder.

6. A number of self-report and interview instruments have proven effective in assessing and diagnosing BPD, including two promising new tools — the McLean Screening Instrument for BPD and the Zanarini Rating Scale for BPD.

7. Factors that indicate increased risk of suicide include lethality of previous attempts, specificity of suicide plans and commitment, availability of the means to commit suicide, impulsivity, substance use, and lack of social support.

8. It is important to differentiate BPD symptoms from those characteristic of other personality disorders, affective disorders, and post-traumatic stress disorder.

# Chapter Three:
# Psychological Approaches to Treating BPD

## This chapter answers the following:

▶ **What are the Various Individual Psychological Approaches to Treating BPD?** — This section focuses on the treatment goals, strategies, and efficacy of the psychodynamic, psychoanalytical, interpersonal, cognitive, dialectical behavior therapy, cognitive analytic, and relapse prevention therapy approaches to treating BPD.

▶ **How Are Various Individual BPD Therapy Approaches Similar?** — This section discusses the five constants of individual BPD psychotherapy.

▶ **How Can Group Psychotherapy Help Those with BPD?** — This section presents an overview of approaches ued in group therapy for those with BPD.

▶ **How Can Psychological Treatment Strategies be used to Manage Suicide Risk?** — This section covers recommendations for managing inpatient care issues, using suicide contracts, psychotherapeutic interventions for suicidal patients, and key issues for clinicians that impact suicide treatment strategies.

RESEARCH supports an environmental influence for BPD through a variety of familial markers (see figure 3.1 below). Such research finds that the majority (up to 91 percent) of people with BPD have experienced significantly higher rates of childhood trauma than non-BPD patients.[78–80] Other research indicates that people with BPD are more likely than those without BPD to report early separation experiences and neglect primarily in the form of emotional withdrawal from early caregivers.[79, 81]

*Families of those with BPD have a higher incidence of borderline-type behaviors, alcoholism, antisocial personality disorder, and other personality disorders.[82–87]*

Additionally, more adults with BPD than those without BPD, experience significantly more violence, such as physical abuse from a partner or recent physical or sexual assault. Four risk factors have been found to predict those with BPD who are adult victims of violence: female gender, substance abuse disorder, childhood sexual abuse, and childhood experience of emotional withdrawal by a caretaker.

*Patients who experienced childhood sexual abuse perpetrated by a parent, tend to engage in more self-destructive behaviors, such as suicide and self-mutilation.[88]*

**Figure 3.1    Familial Markers That Indicate an Environmental Influence for BPD[78, 82]**

| Environmental Influence Factor Reported | % of Those with BPD Reporting each Factor |
|---|---|
| Physical Abuse | 71 |
| Sexual Abuse | 68 |
| Witnessed Serious Domestic Violence | 62 |

# What are the Various Individual Psychotherapeutic Approaches to Treating BPD?

There are numerous theories (many that overlap) regarding the environmental causes of and individual psychological treatments for BPD. The following briefly describes the various environmental theories presented in greater detail later in this chapter.

1. **Psychodynamic Approach** — This approach seeks to produce broad-based character change in which patients gain control of their overwhelming emotions. This control process (also referred to as ego mastery) allows the patients the capacity to form stable relationships and maintain an integrated sense of self.[89]

2. **Psychoanalytic Approach** — Psychoanalytic theorists view BPD as developmental in nature. These theorists believe that people with BPD experienced early trauma that has frustrated or inhibited normal developmental growth. This trauma has kept the person at a "primitive" (or childlike) level of psychic functioning.

3. **Interpersonal Psychotherapy (IPT)** — This approach is based on the theory of personality developed by H.S. Sullivan.[90] This theory defines personality as a relatively enduring pattern of recurrent interpersonal situations. IPT assumes that interpersonal interactions shape current behavior. Consequently, disordered behavior or communications are a result of disordered interpersonal relations.

4. **Cognitive Therapy** — This theory assumes that dysfunction stems from maladaptive *schemas*. These maladaptive schemas result in biased judgments that lead patients to consistently rationalize their own dysfunctional behavior and to be unable to test their interpretations against reality. For example, this approach views people with BPD as holding unrealistic expectations regarding current interpersonal relationships based on rigid beliefs about relationships with early primary caregivers.

5. **Dialectical Behavior Therapy (DBT)** — These theorists stress the relationship between biological and environmental forces. For example, this theory sees the person with BPD as biologically predisposed to being vulnerable to emotional extremes while being influenced by an emotionally invalidating environment.

*IPT's focus on interpersonal interactions presents a marked contrast to the psychoanalytic view that intrapsychic conflicts are expressed on an interpersonal level.*

**schemas** — organized belief systems that attach meaning to events

6. **Cognitive Analytic Therapy** — This section provides a brief overview of a relatively new therapy that helps patients identify and alter reciprocal relationship roles learned through early childhood experiences.

7. **Relapse Prevention** — The relapse prevention model is a social learning model that does not specifically address people with BPD. However, it is a theoretical model for treating people who struggle with addictions. Since people with BPD often have one or more addictions or compulsive behaviors based on immediate gratification, the components of relapse prevention represent important considerations for treatment.

Following the discussion of individual approaches, the section on group psychotherapy provides rationale and benefits for using group therapy with BPD patients rather than specific guidelines on interventions and techniques. The information presented is written for those already experienced in conducting group treatment or those who are planning to refer a patient to group therapy.

## The Psychodynamic Approach to Treating BPD

Psychodynamic approaches seek to help patients gain insight into past unmet emotional needs that influence their currently dysfunctional behavior. These approaches help them identify more direct and appropriate ways to meet their emotional needs. Most psychodynamic approaches focus on the patient's past relationships to help modify current relationships. However, Kernberg et al., who developed the expressive psychotherapy approach, support the primary focus of therapy being on "here-and-now" relationships as a means of interpreting and changing behavior. More traditional psychodynamic approaches focus on the past.[89]

Object relations theorists maintain that the main problem for people with BPD is that they failed to mature psychologically to a point where they can differentiate between self and others. Because they are stuck at this developmental level, BPD patients shift their identity and feelings based on how others react to them. This lack of differentiation of self from others is also related to an inability to balance positive and negative feelings, such as love and aggression.

*Object relations theories represent one school of thought within psychodynamic theories.*

Kernberg et al. attribute this lack of integration of positive and negative feelings to abundant pathological aggression within the BPD patient. This aggression may be biological in nature or it may be a reaction to an early frustrating environment.[39]

## Commonly Used Defense Mechanisms

splitting — the division of
self and others into "all good"
or "all bad" categories, which
results in sudden reversals of
feelings and conceptualizations
about one's self and others

projective identification —
the process whereby the
patient behaves toward
others in such a manner
that elicits the very behavior
that will confirm their own
underlying beliefs

denial — the process
whereby the patient responds
to an event as if it is not or has
not happened

Those with BPD commonly use several defense mechanisms, including *splitting, projective identification,* idealization, and *denial.* These defense mechanisms keep the person with BPD from developing more integrated, useful coping mechanisms. Without these coping mechanisms, the person experiences a general "free floating anxiety," lack of impulse control, and occasional periods of transient psychotic processes.[39]

Splitting happens when people separate themselves and others into "good" and "bad" categories.[86] This view protects BPD sufferers from recognizing their own aggressive impulses. It also allows them to preserve "good" memories of themselves and their primary caregiver rather than feel rage toward their early primary caregiver for not meeting their needs.

Those with BPD who use projective identification, typically elicit the precise behaviors in others that confirm the patients' underlying beliefs. For example, they may accuse the clinician of not caring and not listening. These accusations, usually voiced quite strongly, will likely produce feelings of anger in the clinician. The clinician's angry feelings will then be interpreted by patients as confirmation that the clinician is uncaring, not listening, and not trustworthy to meet their emotional needs.

*The counterpart of idealization
is devaluation, which is the
perception that others are
persecutory or dangerous and
thus completely unable to meet
their needs.*

Idealization allows patients to disavow the clinician's inability to perfectly meet their needs. Because of splitting, patients are unable to recognize that someone who is unable to meet all of their needs can still meet some of their needs.

For BPD patients, denial can be a very strong defense mechanism, strong enough to let patients deny events that they witness. Denial serves the purpose of defending patients' fragile view of themselves and others.

## Treatment Goals and Strategies

The goal of psychodynamic therapy is to help patients identify their feelings (e.g., rage) and identify to what those feelings are a reaction. In this process of identifying the feelings and situation, the patient and clinician can view current events as reflections of past events in which similar needs have gone unmet.

intrapsychic — psychological
processes within a person

*The treatment examples in
figure 3.2 (page 25) demonstrate differences among
traditional, supportive, and
expressive approaches to
psychodynamic treatment.*

Psychodynamic treatment seeks to make characterological changes and assumes that the person's behavior is motivated by *intrapsychic* conflicts that are highly individualized. Psychodynamic methods include **traditional** exploratory, insight-oriented approaches, as well as **supportive** and **expressive** approaches. For each approach, shared views include:

> ▶ The initial therapy session needs to focus on clarifying the role of the clinician and the patient as well as developing a structure for treatment. When the patient

deviates from the therapy contract, there is a framework for interpreting the actions. For example, contracts that call for a commitment to attend therapy sessions provide a groundwork for exploring the feelings and thoughts that led to a particular absence.

▶ To establish vital structure, clinicians must define the limits of their intervention for self-destructive behavior. For example, the clinician may set up a contract with patients that they will seek help at hospital emergency rooms for suicidal or other self-destructive behaviors. (See pages 53–54 for more information on using suicide contracts.)

**Traditional Psychodynamic Treatment** — A leading proponent of exploratory, insight-oriented psychodynamic therapy, W.S. Pollack, has developed a treatment approach that highlights traditional psychodynamic therapy and adds a focus on the developmental process. This integrated developmental-psychodynamic, psychotherapeutic approach includes three phases of treatment:[91]

1. **Holding** — This phase entails helping patients perceive the clinician as a reliable and consistent person who can be depended upon to accept their overt and underlying feelings, including their sadness and rage. BPD patients have not likely experienced a positive, holding relationship in the past and, while they long for such a relationship, they are suspicious of it at the same time. The clinician's ability to empathetically accept this difficulty in trusting will be the most helpful in changing their suspicions. By modifying these suspicions, patients can begin to accept their own ambivalent feelings for the clinician that range from idealization to devastation and rage. The clinician must withstand these extreme emotional expressions and reflect on the loneliness and sense of loss that patients must feel.

2. **Understanding** — This phase requires the clinician to help patients explore their own developmental history and pain. Research indicates that people with BPD often experience very real trauma and abuse as children that affects later adult functioning.[92] Helping patients connect past feelings to their current suspiciousness and feelings increases understanding and decreases the sense of disconnectedness that patients feel with themselves. During this phase, the clinician can help patients understand their behaviors (e.g., dissociation, self-destructive behaviors, rageful enactments) as being functional defense maneuvers they once used to protect themselves.

*Setting up a shared responsibility for therapy sessions and providing a framework for therapy interactions is vital to the success of therapy. To accomplish this shared responsibility, patients must keep track of and relay their own thoughts and feelings related to pertinent impulses and behavior. The clinician then helps them to explore and understand the connection between their thoughts and feelings related to behavior.*

Patients can then come to empathize with their own needs and feel more connected with themselves.

3. **Moving On** — In this phase, the clinician helps patients recognize that they can understand, empathize, and soothe themselves. Additionally, patients become aware that mature interdependence on significant others is necessary for psychological and emotional balance. The clinician supports and encourages patients in this balance of autonomy and affiliation with others.

### Psychodynamic Therapy Efficacy

A randomized controlled study of psychodynamic, group-oriented therapy in a partial hospitalization program yielded positive results. A group of patients with a mixture of personality disorders, including many with BPD, met over the course of 18 weeks. Positive treatment gains included improvements in interpersonal functioning, self-esteem, life satisfaction and defensive functioning that were maintained at the eight-month, follow-up assessment.[93]

Using a structured and manualized form of psychodynamic treatment in an uncontrolled study, researchers found patients who completed the 12-month programs had fewer suicide attempts, fewer hospitalizations, and less severe medical conditions associated with self-injurious behaviors.[94]

## From The Patient's Perspective

*Individual therapy has really helped; now, Owen wants me to do group therapy. I think I will. Alex took our talk well last night. I told her I was angry, and we talked about what happened. I can't believe I was able to talk about my anger rather than go out and pick up someone or cut on myself. I really have made progress. I think group therapy will be helpful too.*

## Figure 3.2   Psychodynamic Treatment Examples (Patient = P  Clinician = C)

$P_1$: Last time we met I could tell you didn't really care about me, you were just seeing me for the money. I was so mad I went home and cut on my wrists. I couldn't help myself.

| Traditional Approach | Supportive Approach | Expressive Approach |
|---|---|---|
| $C_1$: *In what way did it feel like I didn't really care about you?* | $C_1$: *In what way did it feel like I didn't really care about you?* | $C_1$: *In what way did it feel like I didn't really care about you?* |
| $P_2$: When I was talking about my mom being so angry you started taking notes . . . you weren't really listening . . . I'm just another case to you. | $P_2$: When I was talking about my mom being so angry you started taking notes . . . you weren't really listening . . . I'm just another case to you. | $P_2$: When I was talking about my mom being so angry you started taking notes . . . you weren't really listening . . . I'm just another case to you. |
| $C_2$: *You have a lot of strong feelings about this.* | $C_2$: *It sounds like it's very important to you that I care.* | $C_2$: *You have a lot of strong feelings about this.* |
| $P_3$: You bet! I felt so mad. You're supposed to care and listen. I knew all along that you really didn't. | $P_3$: Yeah! When it seemed like you didn't, I just didn't know what to do. It felt like I couldn't go on. You're just interested in my money. | $P_3$: You bet! I felt so mad . . . you're supposed to care and listen. I knew all along that you really didn't. |
| $C_3$: *Is this a familiar feeling?* | $C_3$: *How can you know that I care about you?* | $C_3$: *Is this a familiar feeling?* |
| $P_4$: Yeah, my mom used to ignore me and wouldn't listen. I'd get so mad; it's like I wasn't even there. | $P_4$: I can't; it's clear you don't and never will. | $P_4$: Yeah, my mom used to ignore me and wouldn't listen. I'd get so mad; it's like I wasn't even there. |
| $C_4$: *It sounds like I reminded you of your mom last week?* | $C_4$: *It seems that you really want me to care but it's hard to trust that I do.* | $C_4$: *It sounds like our relationship is very important to you?* |
| $P_5$: Yeah, women really can't be trusted. Men are the only ones that can really be trusted. | $P_5$: Yeah, nobody is trustworthy, everybody abandons me and now you are doing the same. | $P_5$: No, it's not — I used to think it was, but now I know you don't care. |
| $C_5$: *In the past, how did you deal with all that anger about your mom not listening to you?* | $C_5$: *It feels like I'm abandoning you.* | $C_5$: *How did you feel when you thought I didn't care?* |
| $P_6$: I used to just go in my room; I'd be so mad that the only way I could calm myself down was to cut [on wrist and leg]. | $P_6$: Yeah. | $P_6$: I couldn't stand it. I just had to do something. |
| | $C_6$: *I am understanding how important being listened to is to you. It feels like abandonment when you don't feel listened to.* | $C_6$: *So you cut on yourself.* |
| | | $P_7$: Yeah, it makes me feel better. |
| $C_6$: *You did the same thing last week. Sounds like it is very important for you to be listened to.* | $P_7$: Yeah. It feels like I can't trust anybody. | $C_7$: *It sounds like you were angry with me and you took it out on yourself.* |
| $P_7$: Yeah. I hate someone not listening to me. | $C_7$: *That sounds lonely.* | $P_8$: Yeah, cause I know you really don't care to hear about me. |
| | $P_8$: Yeah, now you know why it's so important to me. | $C_8$: *If you were to say to me now what you felt last week when you thought I wasn't listening, what would it be?* |
| $C_7$: *Sounds like you have a hard time sorting me out from your mother.* | | |
| *As the process continues, the client connects early rageful feelings at mother with projecting mother onto the clinician and to current behavior. Alternate response strategies are then explored.* | *Process continues in which the patient feels supported, feelings are reflected, and the relationship is preserved. Through this process, the patient gets help building necessary skills for responding to the sense of abandonment differently next time by talking about their needs and clarifying misunderstandings.* | *The process continues to help the patient disclose feelings, stay focused on the current relationship, and learn how to have a stable relationship with the clinician.* |

## The Psychoanalytic Approach to Treating BPD

Although psychoanalytic theorists represent a school of thought within psychodynamic theories, their therapy focus differs enough to warrant separate reviews. According to these theorists, those with BPD experience early traumas or deficiencies in their environment that lead to a *"psychic deficit."*[95] For people with BPD to protect themselves from the painful awareness of the trauma experienced from their early caregiver, they inhibit their capacity to think about their own as well as others' mental states. This inability to think about the thoughts, feelings, and actions of others and themselves leaves them with overwhelming emotions but no method for processing thoughts about these emotions.

**psychic deficit** — inadequately developed sense of self

People with BPD will often be either *dysphoric* or enraged. This continual emotional oscillation results from dashed hopes for stability and reliable relationships with others, and angry rejection to avoid the personal feelings of aloneness that are so intolerable.[96]

**dysphoric** — generalized feeling of distress

Additionally, research indicates that those with BPD view themselves as hostile, labile, and unstable.[97] Likewise, traditional psychoanalytic theorists maintain that people with BPD primarily defend against primitive aggressive impulses. Because they become easily overwhelmed by these and other emotions, helping them identify and cope with these emotions achieves the main treatment objective of producing basic personality change.

> The main focus of psychoanalytic therapy is to help the person with BPD identify and cope with the aggressive feelings that they work so hard to suppress.

*Pathological internalized object relations* represent the greatest roadblock to effective BPD treatment. Instead of having hope that the clinician will be able to meet their perceived needs, patients' incapacity to tolerate primitive aggression leads to conflict-laden *transference*. These transference feelings result in a deep sense of distrust and fear of the clinician as an "attacker."

**pathological internalized object relations** — extremely dysfunctional relationships with the love objects, which are now carried by the patient as internal beliefs about relationships in general

According to modern psychoanalytic theorists, a traditionally silent response to transference is not beneficial for people with BPD. The clinician needs to combine neutrality with a more active style of doing therapy due to the extreme tendency of those with BPD to misinterpret situations and comments.[95]

**object relations** — present or past relationships with love "objects" — others who are the focus of love or affection

### Treatment Goals and Strategies

Psychoanalysts target seven main goals for therapy:[95]

**transference** — patients respond to clinicians based on particular images of themselves, particular images or beliefs about clinicians, and emotional reactions that connect the two

1. Helping patients integrate their unidentified thoughts and feelings about themselves with their behaviors (reintegrate the split self)

2. Creating an awareness and understanding of patients' object relations and how these affect current behavior

3. Integrating these object relations (the positive and negative aspects, the abilities and inabilities, and the giving and the selfish tendencies) into patients' awareness to help them tolerate their own ambivalent feelings

4. Limiting the patients' acting out of negative impulses, particularly the self-harm impulses, which requires explicit limit setting and establishing consequences for self-destructive behavior (e.g., interpretation, confrontation, suspending a session, enlisting the aid of others, and perhaps even termination of treatment)

5. Promoting higher-level defensive functioning in which the patients' defense mechanisms become part of their awareness and are modified

6. Working through the depression that has resulted from early trauma and abandonment

7. Promoting a sense of the patients' identity being separate from others

> *The clinician must play an active role in repeatedly drawing the patient's attention to the adverse consequences of self-destructive behaviors.*[95]

Like psychodynamic therapy, this theory holds that intrapsychic conflicts are the bases of behavior. There are two general techniques used in psychoanalytic therapy to help define the conflicts. These are maintenance of neutrality and *interpretation*.

**Maintenance of Neutrality** — The clinician must be able to express concern and objectivity in helping patients develop self-understanding without making a personal investment in any one aspect of their behavior. By maintaining this neutrality, the clinician can interpret the needs patients present rather than gratify them. The neutral clinician can calm and support patients and consequently help them to order their internally chaotic world.

> **interpretation** — verbally giving meaning to the link between the patient's unmet needs and current actions

**Interpretation** — To use interpretation, the clinician hypothesizes as to what link exists between the conscious material the patient presents and the patient's unconscious motivations and needs. The clinician then communicates this hypothesis to the patient.[89] Interpretations need to be made to an emotionally prepared patient; therefore, techniques of *clarification* and *confrontation* often precede the use of interpretation.

> **clarification** — exploration of vague or contradictory data
>
> **confrontation** — drawing the patients' attention to data that is discrepant or outside of their awareness

Transference processes are the primary target for interpretation, and the analysis of transference reactions are considered the main vehicle of change. Having the clinician interpret transference helps patients integrate the separate aspects of their feelings and experiences. Interpretation also helps patients sort out reality from distortion in their reactions to the clinician. Additionally, by interpreting both positive and negative impulses toward the clinician, patients can integrate feelings of primitive aggression, which increases their ability to deal with ambivalence.

**regression** — reverting or
retreating into an earlier, more
childlike pattern of behavior

**psychotic transference** —
grossly impaired reality testing
regarding transference issues

For the last several decades, practitioners have exercised cau-tion regarding the use of psychoanalysis to treat those with BPD due to the propensity for *regression* into *psychotic transferences* and uncontrolled acting out. Additionally, some critics of the psychoanalytic approach believe that the emphasis on aggres-sion may leave patients feeling even more critical of themselves for having the aggression. This may negate the possibility that the aggression may result from early environmental trauma and may lead patients to feel responsible for harm perpetrated on them by others.

Figure 3.3, on the next page, illustrates the psychoanalytic approach to the same therapy situation as presented in figure 3.2. This illustration provides a way to compare and contrast the two approaches.

### Psychoanalytic Therapy Efficacy

A randomized, controlled study with severe BPD patients in a partial hospitalization treatment program compared psychoana-lytic treatment to standard psychiatric care over the course of 18 months. The psychoanalytic treatment group received therapy both individually and in a group setting. Psychoanalytic treat-ment produced significantly greater reductions in self mutilating behaviors, suicide attempts, length of inpatient treatment, anxi-ety, and depression as well as improved global adjustment.[98, 99] Further, during the 18 month follow-up period, those from the psychoanlytic group had fewer hospitalizations and emergency room treatments.[100]

Another outcome study focused on the administration of Kohut's self-psychology principles within the psychoanalytic school of thought.[97] The researchers found that following 12 months of individual therapy, there were reductions in impulsivity, affec-tive instability, anger, medical office visits, self-harm behaviors, drug use, and suicidal behavior. However, instead of using a control group as comparison, this study utilized before-and-after survey measures.

The use of long-term treatment techniques is often neither feasible nor appropriate given that most people with BPD fail to complete even six months of treatment.[102]

## Figure 3.3   Psychoanalytic Treatment Example
## (Patient = P    Clinician = C)

$P_1$: **Last time we met I could tell you didn't really care about me, you were just seeing me for the money. I was so mad I went home and cut on my wrists. I couldn't help myself.**

$C_1$: *It seemed like I didn't care.*

$P_2$: Yeah! I know you don't; you never did, you just pretended you did to get my money.

$C_2$: *You sound very angry.*

$P_3$: You bet I am. I can't stand it anymore. I may just go home and end it all because nobody cares.

$C_3$: *It sounds like you are so angry at me you want to get back at me.*

$P_4$: I hate you, you don't hurt like I do, you don't even know what it's like. Everybody leaves me and now you are leaving me too.

$C_4$: *In what way am I leaving you?*

$P_5$: You just don't care, you don't listen. You don't even care that I'm going to go home and kill myself.

$C_5$: *I am noticing that you are angry with me and talking about killing yourself.*

$P_6$: Yeah, I can't stand it anymore.

$C_6$: *What can't you stand?*

$P_7$: You leaving. I knew you would all along.

$C_7$: *I notice that when you talk about leaving and killing yourself that then you say I am leaving.*

$P_8$: I guess it's me who is leaving huh! It just hurts so bad I can't stand it.

$C_8$: *And you feel so mad you want to kill me.*

$P_9$: I didn't say that.

$C_9$: *You are talking about me leaving.*

$P_{10}$: Yeah, but I said I was going to kill myself.

$C_{10}$: *How do you think that is related to killing me?*

$P_{11}$: You said that, I didn't. Anyway, it seems easier to kill myself; it would still end the pain of wanting to kill you.

*The dialog continues to explore the patient's rage toward the clinician and self along with the connection to subsequent behaviors.*

## The Interpersonal Psychotherapy Approach to Treating BPD

The basic premise of interpersonal psychotherapy is that people elicit behavior/communication from others based on a continuous interpersonal negotiation of getting their needs met. This theory assumes that current interpersonal interactions are reactions to earlier experiences in interpersonal relatedness.[90, 103] Further, these interpersonal interactions shape one's self-view and become integrated into one's internal dialogue (self-talk).

Interpersonal theorists maintain that people's rigid and narrow interactions with others cause dysfunctional behavior and communication. Selective attention, wherein people perceive only the information that agrees with and reinforces their particular view, continually reinforces these limited types of interactions. For example, if those with BPD seek nurturing and caring but believe that nobody can really meet their needs (based on earlier interpersonal relations), then they interact with others to make this belief come true. To make this belief come true, they may fail to recognize caring behaviors from others, or they may become easily angered and push others away before their needs are met.

In particular, links between the interpersonal model and BPD include:[105, 106]

1. The patient internalizes abandonment from earlier relationships and behaves very recklessly with self-damaging impulsiveness.

2. Fear of abandonment comes from an early association with trauma and a feeling of self-blame for causing the abandonment. This blaming ("I'm a bad person.") results from punitive interactions with primary caregivers.

3. Internalization of neglect and its association with boredom and loneliness lead to feelings of emptiness.

4. Instability results from chaotic, early familial interactions that had serious consequences.

5. Those with BPD exhibit intense anger set off by perceived abandonment that is intended to coerce the opposite of abandonment, namely nurturance.

6. Self-mutilation can be a replay of early abuse from caregivers or an effort to appease an internalized attacker (negative internal message). Additionally, research indicates that those with BPD who engage in self-mutilating behaviors have poorer skills in communicating non-verbal emotional information to others and in interpreting such information from others.[107]

*One interpersonal theorist describes all human experience as an internal dialogue or communication with other persons, whether imaginary or real; accordingly, a person's self has no existence apart from relationships with other persons.[104]*

*Within this model, psychiatric diagnoses of personality disorders can be made based on patterns of maladaptive interactions.[105]*

7. Identity disturbance stems from the internalization of early caregivers, who would attack the person with BPD when there were signs of independence, self-definition, and/or happiness.

8. Self-sabotage amounts to self-protection from internalized abusers.

9. Thought disorder or poor reality perception may result from negated reality testing in earlier interpersonal interactions.

## Treatment Goals and Strategies

Interpersonal psychotherapy treatment methods use a *collaborative* manner and focus on identifying self-defeating communication styles, clarifying reactions, and establishing alternatives to maladaptive behavior. In this approach, there are three main treatment goals:

1. **Identifying self-defeating communication styles** — Identifying these styles requires recognizing that patients will send the same rigid and self-defeating messages to the clinician that they send to others.

2. **Clarifying reactions** — Once the clinician is aware of the "pulls" and "tugs" to respond to a patient in a certain manner, the clinician needs to purposefully not respond that way. Instead, the clinician poses hypotheses to the patient about the effects of such interactions. Additionally, one of the most powerful forms of therapeutic change is for clinicians to respond to the patient in a very genuine manner that clarifies their own "pulls" (reactions) to the patient.

3. **Establishing alternatives** — The goal during this phase is to help patients establish alternate patterns to previous maladaptive interpersonal patterns. The clinician and patients analyze the previous patterns of interaction that have produced undesirable results. They then discuss alternates. For example, if a patient has a pattern of responding passively during an interaction and then later becoming angry and engaging in self-harm behavior, then the clinician will help the patient engage in alternate, more active response patterns.

**collaborative** — clinician and patient putting equal effort toward agreed-upon goals

*The treatment example in figure 3.4, on page 32, demonstrates how the interpersonal clinician might respond to the same initial patient comment used in the other examples.*

**Figure 3.4    Interpersonal Therapy Treatment Example
(Patient = P    Clinician = C)**

$P_1$: **Last time we met I could tell you didn't really care about me, you were just seeing me for the money. I was so mad I went home and cut on my wrists. I couldn't help myself.**

$C_1$: *You feel that I don't care.*

$P_2$: I know you don't, you proved that last week!

$C_2$: *Can you help me understand your anger?*

$P_3$: What do you mean help you understand? You're supposed to care, you're my therapist.

$C_3$: *You want me to care.*

$P_4$: Damn right I do — but I know you don't really.

$C_4$: *It is important to you that I care and yet when I am angrily accused of not caring, I feel the pull to be more distant rather than to come closer and be more caring.*

$P_5$: So you don't care. I knew it all along.

$C_5$: *I am saying that you are asking for my caring and closeness in a way that makes me feel pushed away rather than close.*

$P_6$: *So . . . I'm angry at you for not caring and you're saying it's my fault?*

$C_6$: *I'm wondering how we can resolve this in a way that you find out what you want, and we are closer rather than more distant.*

$P_7$: What I want is to know if you care or not?

$C_7$: *How can you find that out from me without pushing me away?*

$P_8$: Well, I guess I could tell you how your taking notes last week made me feel and see if you meant it that way?

$C_8$: *How would that be different than what you have already done?*

$P_9$: Well, I guess I wouldn't just be accusing you, which you say makes you want to be more distant.

$C_9$: *Yes. It sounds like this approach will be different for you.*

$P_{10}$: Yeah, I'm used to just letting people know how angry I am.

$C_{10}$: *Do you get the kind of response you want from them?*

$P_{11}$: Well, they always prove me right!

$C_{11}$: *They prove you right?*

$P_{12}$: Yeah, I tell them I'm mad, and tell them why. Then, they can't handle it and go away.

$C_{12}$: *So they become more distant instead of working out the problem with you.*

$P_{13}$: Yeah, maybe it's kind of like what you were saying you feel . . . more distant.

## Interpersonal Therapy Efficacy

The recently published interpersonal treatment approach outlined in the System for Classifying Interpersonal Behavior (SASB) lacks the supportive research to substantiate its effectiveness in treating BPD or other personality disorders. However, researchers utilized a more general type of interpersonal psychotherapy in treating BPD and compared it to other treatments, including cognitive-behavioral therapy.[108] Results found cognitive-behavioral therapy to be superior to interpersonal therapy over a 16-week period for people with BPD.

## The Cognitive Approach to Treating BPD

This theory assumes that the event itself doesn't lead to a particular consequence; it's the person's belief about the event that gives it meaning and relates it to subsequent behavior. For example, high winds and dark clouds don't in themselves lead someone to run for cover. It is people's beliefs that these weather patterns result in tornados that lead them to seek shelter.

In the **Cognitive Therapy of Personality Disorders**, Beck relates that personality disorders are dysfunctions largely due to certain schemas that lead to biased judgments.[109] These dysfunctional schemas lead people to consistently create erroneous beliefs and interpretations of their own as well as others' actions, which leads to dysfunctional emotion and behavior.

Cognitive theorists view people with BPD as having extreme and poorly integrated views of relationships with early caregivers (similar to the object relations view). As a result, they hold extreme, unrealistic expectations regarding current interpersonal relationships. These expectations shape their behavioral and emotional responses and account for many BPD symptoms.

Beck proposes three basic assumptions underlying the perceptions and interpretations of a person with BPD.[109] These are:

1. **"The world is dangerous and malevolent."** — This perception leads to the conclusion that taking risks is dangerous. These risks include letting down one's guard, revealing a personal weakness, or being "out of control." Such beliefs lead to chronic feelings of tension, tiredness, suspicion, and guardedness.

2. **"I am powerless and vulnerable."** — This perception leads people with BPD to believe that they cannot deal with the dangerous and malevolent world they view. Patients typically resolve this dilemma by becoming dependent upon someone they see as capable of taking care of them. However, people with BPD find this dependence unacceptable because they believe they are inherently unlovable and unacceptable.

*Nine Common Maladaptive Schemas Characteristic of Those with BPD*[96, 110]

1. *Abandonment/Loss* — "I'll be alone; no one will be there for me."

2. *Unlovability* — "No one would love me if they really got to know me."

3. *Dependence* — "I can't cope on my own; I need someone to rely on."

4. *Subjugation/Lack of Individuation* — "If I don't do what others want, they'll abandon me or attack me."

5. *Mistrust* — "People will hurt me, attack me, or take advantage of me. I must protect myself."

6. *Inadequate Self/Discipline* — "I can't control myself."

7. *Fear of Losing Emotional Control* — "I must control my emotions or something terrible will happen."

8. *Guilt/Punishment* — "I'm a bad person. I deserve to be punished."

9. *Emotional Deprivation* — "No one is ever there to meet my needs or to care for me."

**3. "I am inherently unacceptable."** — This belief keeps people with BPD from trusting others to maintain a relationship once that person "really gets to know me." Another common type of cognitive distortion in which people with BPD commonly engage involves overshadowing high-achieving activities with the belief that, "I am a fake; someday, they will find me out."

An important goal of therapy is to help patients with BPD evaluate and modify their *dichotomous thinking*.[109] These extreme interpretations of events lead to extreme emotional responses and actions. With this type of thinking, there are no categories for intermediate perceptions. Therefore, the person with BPD may initially perceive others as reliable and completely trustworthy until the first time they fall short. At that point, they will be seen as completely untrustworthy. Dichotomous thinking precludes the idea that people may be trustworthy most of the time or in most situations.

Because dichotomous thinking causes patients with BPD to view themselves as either flawless or completely unacceptable, they see shortcomings in themselves as evidence that they are completely unacceptable as a person. Therefore, those with BPD feel they must hide these shortcomings from others. Consequently, they must avoid intimacy and openness in a relationship for fear they will be "found out." By not getting needed closeness and security from a relationship, they will typically experience feelings of hopelessness. This self-reinforcing cycle is often quite resistant to change.

One of the goals of cognitive therapy is to help patients test their underlying beliefs and modify them to bring about desired changes. This cognitive shift changes dysfunction-causing beliefs into an anxiety state necessary for change and, ultimately, into more functional belief systems.

### Treatment Goals and Strategies

Beck outlines eight intervention strategies for treating the person with BPD using a cognitive theoretical approach.[109] These are:

**1. Develop trust in the relationship and use a collaborative strategy** — Establishing the clinician/patient relationship in and of itself challenges most of the assumptions held by those with BPD. A trusting relationship can most easily be established when the clinician openly acknowledges how difficult it must be for patients to trust based on the number of painful experiences they have had in the past. Then, the clinician must behave in a consistently trustworthy manner by only making promises that can be kept and by carefully defining the relationship so that patients know what to expect.

---

**dichotomous thinking** — tendency to perceive and characterize situations, others' actions, and solutions as "black or white," "all or nothing," "good or bad," "trustworthy or deceitful," "successful or complete failures"

*The conflict between wanting to have someone to depend on and feeling inherently unacceptable causes the person with BPD to vacillate radically between autonomy and dependence, without being able to rely on either for emotional support.*

*Cognitive theorists see changing dysfunctional beliefs in people with personality disorders as more difficult than in others due to inherently greater levels of extremes and rigid beliefs.*

*Building a collaborative relationship is often a slow process even though it is an important treatment factor.*

2. **Choose an initial focus of therapy with the patient that will lead to some immediately felt progress** — Behavioral goals can often be useful at this point in therapy because they take the focus off of the difficulties involved in maintaining trust and intimacy.

3. **Reduce or eliminate dichotomous thinking early in therapy** — As the main contributor to extreme actions, mood swings, and dilemmas faced by those with BPD, reducing dichotomous thinking should reduce symptom intensity as well as help modify underlying assumptions and provide alternate resolutions to many dilemmas. To change dichotomous thinking, the clinician should point out examples to the patient as they occur and then using the same example to help the patient identify a variety of different perspectives that would lead to more realistic and adaptive responses.

4. **Deal with the transference issues in the session** — Transference can best be understood in cognitive terms as patients responding to the clinician based on generalized beliefs and expectations they have about relationships, rather than according to how the clinician behaves as an individual. When strong emotional reactions occur that appear to be related to transference reactions, the clinician must deal with them promptly. Cognitive treatment practitioners suggest the following process:

   > *Transference reactions are a very rich source of material for uncovering dysfunctional thoughts and assumptions.*

   ▶ Develop a clear understanding of what the patient is thinking and feeling.

   ▶ Resolve misunderstandings and misconceptions clearly and explicitly.

   ▶ Convey that the patient will not be rejected or attacked because of emotional reactions.

5. **Address the patient's fear of change directly by examining the risks involved in trying things a new way** — One perception common among people with BPD that is based on fear of change is that therapy will end once they overcome their problems. If this is the case, the clinician needs to clarify that termination of therapy will be a collaborative decision as will other decisions about therapy.

6. **Help patients increase control over their emotions by acknowledging their emotions and modeling appropriate ways to respond to them** — The clinician can help patients look critically at their thoughts in a problem situation and develop alternate coping strategies. These strategies involve learning adaptive ways to express emotions. While developing these more active and assertive responses, the clinician should proceed

slowly and should continue to talk about the risks in changing behavior patterns. For example, many people with BPD believe expressing anger will lead to immediate rejection or attack by the recipient.

7. **Improve impulse control by acknowledging and dealing with the patient's initial response to changing behavior, "Why should I?"** — Most people with BPD have been told numerous times that they should better control themselves. As a result, they will likely oppose behavior change. Clinicians need to convey to patients that they are not trying to enforce societal norms, but that they are helping them choose whether to act on an impulse or not. The process of developing impulse control involves:

   ▸ Identifying impulses

   ▸ Exploring the pros and cons of controlling impulses

   ▸ Developing alternatives to responding to impulses

   ▸ Examining the expectations and fears that block promising alternatives

   ▸ Providing skills training or coaching necessary for the patient to utilize new alternatives

*In choosing whether to act on an impulse, the patient will not necessarily need to behave in ways they may later regret.*

Additionally, the clinician needs to discuss what the impulse behavior means to the patient as well as the motivation for performing that behavior. For example, self-mutilation acts may come from a desire to punish others, punish oneself, obtain relief from guilt, or as a distraction from more aversive thoughts and feelings. Knowing the motivation behind the behavior can help in developing alternate coping strategies.

8. **Strengthen the patient's sense of identity** — Help patients identify their positive characteristics and accomplishments and provide them with positive feedback regarding their resourceful decisions and effective coping. In addition, have them evaluate their own actions realistically as a means of strengthening their own ability to provide positive self-reinforcement. The patient/clinician relationship presents the single most important opportunity for providing positive feedback; the clinician can provide positive feedback to the patient by recognizing difficult risks the patient takes in therapy.

Figure 3.5, below, demonstrates how the clinician using cognitive therapy might respond to the same initial comment as used in previous examples.

**Figure 3.5   Cognitive Therapy Treatment Example
(Patient = P    Clinician = C)**

$P_1$: **Last time we met I could tell you didn't really care about me, you were just seeing me for the money. I was so mad I went home and cut on my wrists. I couldn't help myself.**

$C_1$: *It sounds like you were very angry.*

$P_2$: You bet I was. I knew you didn't care about me all along.

$C_2$: *What were you feeling when you decided to cut on yourself?*

$P_3$: I already told you, I was very angry with you.

$C_3$: *When you were feeling angry, what were you thinking?*

$P_4$: I was thinking that life was hopeless, nobody would ever care about me. Not even you.

$C_4$: *You were thinking that nobody cares about you and never will in the future?*

$P_5$: Kinda like that.

$C_5$: *Well I can see why you felt hopeless. I believe I would too if nobody cared about me, and nobody ever would in the future. That sounds pretty lonely. What kept you from killing yourself?*

$P_6$: Well it wasn't bad enough to kill myself.

$C_6$: *What do you mean it wasn't "bad enough"?*

$P_7$: Well, I was really mad at you. I guess I didn't really think "nobody" cares. If nobody cared, I think I would kill myself.

$C_7$: *There are some people in your life that care about you?*

$P_8$: Yeah, I guess.

$C_8$: *How do you know when someone cares about you.*

$P_9$: Well they listen to me, and talk to me, and help me.

$C_9$: *Who do you know who listens to you and talks to you?*

$P_{10}$: Well, my friend Trudy does.

$C_{10}$: *How well does she do? Is she pretty good at being able to listen to you most of the time?*

$P_{11}$: Yes, she's always there when I need her. I can always count on her.

$C_{11}$: *That's pretty amazing that she is always there. Most friends are able to be there a lot of the time, but not all of the time.*

$P_{12}$: Well yes, I guess she's not there all the time, but most of the time.

By admitting that a significant relationship is not "perfect," the clinician continues to bring the discussion back to the current relationship with the clinician. The goal is to help the patient acknowledge feelings of wanting the clinician to "always" be attentive and "perfect," but let the patient know the clinician cares and will be there but not "always" or "perfectly." This technique helps the patient identify the ability to have a "non-perfect" caring relationship in a less threatening way and then transfer that understanding to the current therapeutic relationship.

## Cognitive Therapy Efficacy

*Feedback by the clinician must be provided in an honest and realistic manner so that it does not appear insincere.*

There are few controlled outcome studies assessing the efficacy of cognitive therapy with BPD. However, one study completed by the National Institute of Mental Health found cognitive-behavioral therapy to be superior to interpersonal therapy over a 16-week period for treating people with BPD.[108]

## The Dialectical Behavior Therapy Approach to Treating BPD

**dialectical** — systematic reasoning processes where a person tries to resolve contradictory ideas

*Dialectical* behavior therapy (DBT) is an approach originally developed by Linehan to treat suicidal behaviors.[111-114] This approach, which has been expanded to treat people with BPD, focuses on the inherent tension between often-opposing forces. For example, on one hand, the clinician needs to initiate change in the patient and, on the other hand, the clinician must demonstrate acceptance of the patient as they are "in the moment." Both forces are critical to the BPD treatment and highlight the dialectical bases of treatment.

**emotional dysregulation** — emotional imbalance or poor emotional control

DBT is based on a long-term treatment model that views BPD in a biosocial model. The theory proposes that those with BPD have a biological predisposition toward *emotional dysregulation* coupled with an emotionally invalidating environment.[115, 116] These forces interact to produce the dysfunction seen in BPD.

DBT focuses on three sets of opposing forces that clarify primary BPD conflicts:

**blocking** — disruption or inhibition of thought processes

1. **Emotional vulnerability vs. self-invalidation** — The emotional vulnerability syndrome refers to the poor ability that many people with BPD have in regulating their emotions. They are extremely sensitive to even low-level emotional stimuli. They tend to react quickly and have more intense responses to emotions than others. Additionally, they return more slowly to their own emotional baseline, consequently they will often go to great lengths to avoid emotions by using denial, avoidance, *blocking*, and shutting down. When unable to avoid emotion, they intensely overreact with extreme emotional displays or engage in various dysfunctional escape behaviors, such as substance abuse and/or other self-harm behaviors. Some research indicates that this type of emotional sensitivity is constitutional in nature.[117]

   The self-invalidation syndrome describes the discounting of personal feelings. Those with BPD often grew up in environments where feelings were negated or not addressed. As a result, they failed to learn how to accept, label, or control their own feelings.[118]

Vulnerability to extreme emotions, coupled with the lack of validation for these emotions, leads the person to feel guilty, overwhelmed, and afraid that their emotions are uncontrollable.

2. **Unrelenting crises vs. inhibited grieving** — Those with BPD often live in a perpetual state of crisis, while desperately trying to avoid or inhibit feelings of grief that result from the crises. *Unrelenting crisis* refers to the repeated emotional reactivity experienced by the person with BPD. Intense emotional reactions increase distress because they interfere with the ability to plan behaviors as well as to think clearly and solve problems. Because the ability to tolerate one's own emotions is so low, those with BPD often engage in counterproductive escape behaviors, such as drinking, spending money, engaging in unprotected sex, and leaving situations, which creates more losses and crises.

**unrelenting crisis** — the individual does not return to an emotional baseline before the next crisis hits

Inhibited grieving syndrome refers to a pattern of recurrent loss as a result of the many crises created by unpredictable behavior and emotional stress. Crisis of any kind involves loss, whether it be concrete — the loss of a job, a significant other, a predictable environment — or abstract — the loss of acceptance by someone. The loss is not experienced and grieved due to the poor ability to deal with emotions. This creates a perpetual system of *bereavement overload.*[119]

3. **Active passivity vs. apparent competence** — *Active passivity* refers to the tendency of those with BPD to demand that their difficulties be resolved by others in their environment. The passivity stems from a sense of hopelessness because the individual has learned few coping responses and cannot avoid extreme negative emotions. This hopelessness often leads to interpersonal dependency marked by emotional clinging and demanding behaviors.

**bereavement overload** — overwhelming number of feelings related to grief and loss

**active passivity** — the tendency to approach problems in a passive and helpless manner

The *apparent competency syndrome* highlights how those with BPD may mask their true feelings or adopt the attitude of others, even in painful situations. This often results in patients appearing very competent in a particular situation, while later displaying extreme negative emotions to the bewilderment of those around them. Thus, the person may behave appropriately and competently in one situation, which gives observers the false impression that they are able to act competently across many situations.

**apparent competency syndrome** — the tendency to appear deceptively competent

### DBT Behavioral Targets

1. Decrease suicide behaviors

2. Decrease behaviors that interfere with therapy

3. Decrease behaviors that interfere with quality of life, such as substance abuse, homelessness, joblessness, or poor relationship abilities

4. Increase coping skills of emotional regulation, distress tolerance, and interpersonal skills

5. Decrease post-traumatic stress responses through accepting and changing current patterns between thoughts, feelings, and behaviors

6. Enhance self-respect

7. Focus on achieving individual patient goals

## Treatment Goals and Strategies

DBT involves four primary stages of treatment: overall stabilization, helping patients heal the effects of trauma, addressing residual problems that interfere with achieving personal goals, and helping patients resolve feelings of incompleteness. Within these stages, patients focus on seven main dialectical forces (detailed in figure 3.6 on the next page), and clinicians use six primary types of treatment strategies (discussed on pages 41 through 43).[11, 112, 113]

### Stages of Treatment

**Stage 1: Overall stabilization — treatment goals:**

- Decreasing life-threatening behaviors, such as suicide, unprotected sex, and substance abuse
- Increasing connections to supportive individuals, such as family members, clinician, and close friends
- Reinforcing stability, capabilities, and control of action to achieve goals, including increasing skills in:
  - Interpersonal effectiveness
  - Distress tolerance (e.g., feeling and respecting emotional discomfort)
  - Objective thinking (e.g., observing, describing, taking a non-judgmental stance)
  - Being effective with one thing in the moment

**Stage 2: Helping patients heal the effects of trauma in their lives — treatment goals:**

- Understanding early trauma, such as neglect and physical/sexual assaults and reducing counterproductive avoidance behaviors
- Increasing productive connections to people, places, and activities, such as supportive family and friends and work

**Stage 3: Addressing residual problems that interfere with achieving personal goals — treatment goal:** Focusing on behavior patterns that increase self-respect and self-trust

**Stage 4: Helping patients resolve feelings of incompleteness and increasing their capacity for sustained joy — treatment goals:**

- Setting additional personal goals
- Expanding awareness and spiritual fulfillment

*Areas of Focus for Patients*

The seven, main opposing forces or dialectical areas of focus for patients are explained in figure 3.6 below.

### Figure 3.6 DBT Focus Areas

| Patients Focus on Balancing . . . | | |
|---|---|---|
| **Self acceptance and problem acceptance** — Acceptance of one's own strengths, weaknesses and problems to decrease guilt, shame, and distress | *vs.* | **Improving one's effectiveness and problem solving** — actively engaging in skill building and problem solving to initiate change |
| **Tolerating emotions** — Increase ability to tolerate uncomfortable and painful emotions to reduce counterproductive avoidance behaviors (e.g., self-mutilation, shutting off feelings, leaving situations) | *vs.* | **Regulating and controlling emotions** — Regulating and controlling overwhelming emotions through specific distraction or self-soothing strategies |
| **Seeking help and depending on others** — Needing and relying on others for support and help | *vs.* | **Independence and self-efficacy** — Believing in one's own independent abilities and personally taking care of problems or dilemmas |
| **Focusing on others** — Increasing one's ability to attend to other peoples' thoughts and feelings (as well as one's own)* | *vs.* | **Focusing on self** — Feeling better about one's self by focusing on and giving to other people, which improves relationships |
| **Participating effectively** — Identifying ways to control or change a situation through effective participation | *vs.* | **Attending and watching** — Observing and watching how events unfold, developing reflection and impulse-control skills to increase planned behavior |
| **Revealing one's self to others** — Deciding which personal thoughts and feelings to share with others to build relationships | *vs.* | **Retaining privacy** — Determining thoughts and feelings to keep private to increase self-respect and healing |
| **Trusting others** — Identifying specific characteristics or circumstances with others that can be trusted | *vs.* | **Suspecting Others** — Deciding what characteristics/circumstances one should be suspicious about** |

\* Because of their high levels of emotional discomfort, those with BPD tend to be very self-focused.

\*\*Finding a balance between trust and suspicion encourages more reflective and moderate interactions with others.

*Treatment Strategies for Clinicians*

DBT uses six specific strategies — dialectical, focus on commitment, validation, problem-solving, reciprocal and irreverent communication, and case management.[11, 112, 113]

1. **Dialectical strategies** — These strategies, including the use of stories, myths, and paradoxes, focus on helping the patient balance cognitive and emotional extremes as well as use their *wise mind.*

   The clinician focuses on primary opposing forces to help patients find interpersonal, emotional, and cognitive balance.

**wise mind** — the part of the person that pays attention and attaches meaning to all that is happening around them

**The main dialectical strategies during treatment sessions include:**

- ▶ Alternating acceptance and change strategies to encourage a collaborative working alliance
- ▶ Balancing nurturing and accepting responses with demands for the patients to actively change or help themselves
- ▶ Focusing on patient capabilities as well as on personal limitations and deficits
- ▶ Modeling critical and observational thinking by focusing on patients' viewpoints as well as other perspectives or missing information
- ▶ Describing and encouraging flexibility and change on a developmental level, while acknowledging patient needs for stability
- ▶ Synthesizing apparently opposite thoughts and feelings to help patients identify the middle path inherent in all aspects of life

*The clinician must convey that the change-making process consists of taking small steps toward a larger goal rather than trying to change too quickly.*

2. **Focusing on commitment** — Clinicians ask the patient to commit to small, initial changes before eventually asking for larger commitments to change. Likewise, they approach commitment by asking for more than the patient will give, and then reducing the request until the patient commits. These strategies focus on getting the patient to commit to changes that reinforce adaptive, non-suicidal behavior and extinguish maladaptive and suicidal behaviors.

*The therapy relationship is best for challenging the assumption that, "I am inherently unacceptable." The clinician challenges this assumption through honestly appreciating patients for who they are and helping them perceive themselves as acceptable.*

3. **Validation strategies** — These strategies focus on accepting, empathizing with, and reflecting on the patient's behaviors and feelings in light of present circumstances. This process involves:

- ▶ Discovering and helping the patient understand how current behavior protects them from something painful
- ▶ Perpetually putting forth the belief that the patient wants to improve (requires the clinician to acknowledge how feelings of shame, fear, and anger may inhibit improvement)

**contingency** — an agreement between the clinician and patient regarding specific behaviors that will be followed by specific reinforcers or punishers

4. **Problem-solving strategies** — Problem-solving strategies focus on change. Once the clinician and patient identify a problem behavior, skills training can be used to increase coping capabilities; cognitive strategies can be used to modify beliefs, rules, and expectancies; and *contingency* management can be used to increase incentives for adaptive coping.

5. **Reciprocal and irreverent communication strategies** — These strategies seek to interweave communication of warmth, acceptance, and closeness with a matter-of-fact approach and confrontation. The clinician uses self-disclosure to model coping skills and encourage self-disclosure by the patient. Irreverent communication strategies balance clinician responses of warmth and acceptance with the introduction of more offbeat responses to maladaptive behaviors. These offbeat responses may help "unbalance" the patient, creating a shift that promotes acceptance of a new viewpoint. If used carefully, this strategy can facilitate problem solving without the risk that excessive attention may reinforce suicidal or escape behaviors.

6. **Case management strategies** — These strategies balance the clinician's need to provide environmental interventions in situations where immediate outcomes are very important, with consultant-to-the-patient strategies that encourage patients to act on their own behalf. Additionally, the clinician can use self-supervision/consultation to balance the tension between caring for one's self and caring for the patient.

*The clinician must neither reinforce suicidal behavior through excessive attention nor ignore these behaviors to the point that the patient escalates them to a life-threatening level.*

*The treatment example in figure 3.7, on the following page, demonstrates how the clinician using DBT strategies might help validate the patient's feelings and support the development of alternate behaviors. Compare this example with the previous treatment examples; all respond to the same initial comment by the patient.*

## DBT Efficacy

In randomized, controlled studies comparing DBT to "treatment as usual" (TAU), DBT outcome was found to be superior to TAU in the community as measured by:[120–124]

- ► Fewer self-damaging, impulsive behaviors
- ► Fewer severe borderline symptoms
- ► Greater gains in global and social adjustment
- ► Fewer parasuicidal behaviors
- ► Fewer inpatient hospitalizations
- ► Lower attrition rates
- ► Less medically severe parasuicides following one year of therapy

Other non-controlled studies found DBT superior to "treatment as usual in the community" in terms of patients reporting significantly less anger, greater social adjustment, better work performance, less anxious rumination, and feeing less severely disturbed following one year of therapy.[126, 129]

*Other non-controlled studies found DBT superior to "treatment as usual in the community" in terms of patients reporting significantly less anger, greater social adjustment, better work performance, less anxious rumination, and feeling less severely disturbed following one year of therapy.[125, 126]*

*In these efficacy studies, patients who were randomly assigned to the "treatment as usual in the community" group received treatment from various community professionals, most of whom reported that they practiced behavioral or cognitive-behavioral therapy.*

**Figure 3.7    Dialectical Behavior Therapy Treatment
Example (Patient = P    Clinician = C)**

$P_1$: **Last time we met I could tell you didn't really care about me,
you were just seeing me for the money. I was so mad I went
home and cut on my wrists. I couldn't help myself.**

$C_1$: *What made it seem like I didn't care?*

$P_2$: You started taking notes when I was telling you how angry I was
with my mother.

$C_2$: *When I wrote some notes that meant that I didn't care about you?*

$P_3$: Right, that you weren't really listening to me.

$C_3$: *I can understand how my looking away from you in order to write a
note seemed as if I wasn't listening. I am sorry that it came across that
way and you felt discounted.*

$P_4$: Yeah, well!

$C_4$: *I'm wondering when you became aware of feeling angry?*

$P_5$: Right away. I just didn't say anything.

$C_5$: *So when you went home and cut on yourself that was your way of
stopping the angry feelings?*

$P_6$: Yes, and it worked for a while.

$C_6$: *I'm wondering how you can honor your angry feelings without cutting
on yourself.*

$P_7$: Honor my anger?

$C_7$: *Right. Your feelings are important.*

$P_8$: Well, that seems like a joke, but I guess I could tell you when
I'm angry.

$C_8$: *How will that help you know that I'm listening and I care about you?*

$P_9$: I guess if you quit taking notes or something.

$C_9$: *We could figure out another method for remembering important things
you say.*

$P_{10}$: Hum, well I guess we could come up with something. Honoring my
anger! That sure is different. My anger doesn't seem so unbearable
when I look at it like that.

*The dialog continues with focus on helping the patient tolerate uncomfort-
able angry feelings as well as problem solve regarding note taking.*

*Chapter four covers
medications used to treat
BPD, including SSRIs (selective
serotonin reuptake inhibitors)
and atypical antipsychotics.*

Randomized controlled trials have evaluated the effectiveness
of DBT with and without combined medication therapy, compared to placebo. In one study, DBT was superior to placebo
in reducing depression, anxiety, anger, and dissociation. DBT
combined with fluoxetine treatment (an SSRI medication), did
not show any advantages over DBT alone.[127] However, combined
treatment of DBT with olanzapine (an atypical antipsychotic
medication), proved superior to placebo in reducing depression,
anxiety, and impulsive aggressive behavior.[128]

## The Cognitive Analytic Therapy Approach to Treating BPD

Cognitive analytic therapy — a newly developed, brief integrative treatment model — focuses on learned patterns of relating to others. This developmental model emphasizes early childhood experiences and learned relationship roles that are the focus of treatment. Patients learn to recognize their repertoire of *reciprocal roles* so that they may decide how to revise their behavior to be more functional and adaptive. Additionally, emphasis is placed on strengthening awareness and control of the dissociative process that occurs in many with BPD.[130] Preliminary research on the effectiveness of this approach is promising.[130-136]

**reciprocal roles** — thoughts and actions directed toward eliciting or predicting a particular response

## The Relapse Prevention Therapy Approach to Treating BPD

In relapse prevention therapy, the overall aim is to teach the patient how to achieve a *balanced lifestyle* and to prevent unhealthy habit patterns by anticipating and coping with relapse.[137] By acquiring new skills and cognitive strategies, the patient can regulate new behaviors with higher mental processes including awareness and responsible decision-making. However, this process requires the patient to take an active position toward mastering new skills. This is problematic for people with BPD until their characteristic passive stance has been sufficiently moderated. In this model, clinicians view addictive behavior as an acquired habit pattern rather than as a disease.

**balanced lifestyle** — a lifestyle in which the patient has control of their behavior and chooses generally moderate behaviors

One of the main assumptions of this theory is that factors associated with the initial development of an addictive behavior may be independent of factors associated with changing that behavior. For example, the initial development of alcoholism may be the result of a genetic aberration or of an unbalanced metabolic system. Based on this etiology, some would expect a change in drinking behavior to be brought about only through a biomedical intervention. Instead, relapse prevention therapy strives to help patients master the skills necessary to live the life they desire.

To better understand addiction, both clinician and patient should know that addictive actions are usually followed by some form of immediate gratification (e.g., a high state of pleasure or tension reduction), which increases the desire to repeat the behavior. However, these behaviors are unhealthy to the extent that they lead to delayed but negative social, health, and/or self-esteem consequences.

The relapse prevention model supports the view that uncontrollable addictive behaviors are cyclical in nature. Figure 3.8, on the following page, illustrates how this cycle works.

*Relapse prevention is a theoretical model for treating people who struggle with addictions. Since people with BPD often have one or more addictions or compulsive behaviors based on immediate gratification, the components of relapse prevention represent important treatment considerations.*

## Figure 3.8    Cycle of Addictive Behavior

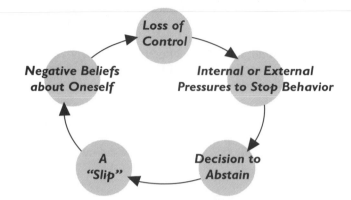

The goal of relapse prevention therapy is to help patients be aware of their behavior, choose skills appropriate to the situation, and follow a behavior course that is midway between restraint and indulgence.

The relapse prevention model for treating addiction requires active patient participation in changing behavior. The model proposes three stages of change:

1. **Motivation and commitment** — Motivation to change may come from an individual desire, an awareness of long-term negative consequences, failure to derive desired beneficial effects, or confrontation from others. After determining the patient's motivation, both clinician and patient need to discuss commitment to change and the patient's sense of timing and lifestyle. If this commitment is not carefully considered, an impulsive attempt to change based on the motivation may fail, which makes a patient reluctant to recommit to the change process.

2. **Implementation** — This stage utilizes behavioral, cognitive, and lifestyle interventions targeted toward changing from a maladaptive pattern of responding to a more purposeful response pattern.

3. **Maintenance** — This stage is the most difficult and needs the most attention. Maintenance begins the moment abstinence or control begins. Because this is the stage in which patients will be faced with multiple temptations, they need planned strategies to cope with these urges. Old, problematic habits must be "unlearned," and new behaviors must be acquired. Most *mistakes* are likely to occur during this stage as patients gradually learn new replacement behaviors. These mistakes

*Though this is a learning model, the assumption is not that the person is solely responsible for their addictions. Rather, addictions are viewed as a result of behavioral reinforcement of which the person is usually unaware.*

**mistakes** — recurrences of behaviors being "unlearned" and framed as mistakes to be learned from subside as patients master new response patterns. These mistakes are considered *lapses*, while a total reversal to the old behavior patterns is considered a *relapse*.

Clinicians give lapses and relapses a framework, allowing patients to view them as a way to learn how to make new behavior patterns work. In these instances, it may be better to term the slip as a *prolapse* to suggest working toward an overall beneficial outcome.

Because patients' negative emotional states (e.g., anger, sadness, frustration, and feelings of abandonment) have been involved in 35 percent of relapses, the clinician should assess with the patient the main sources of negative (unpleasant) emotional reactions.[137] These sources include:

▶ Various interpersonal interactions

▶ Negative self-image

▶ Learned beliefs that cause distressful emotional reactions

## Treatment Goals and Strategies

Relapse prevention involves six, key treatment approaches:

1. **Taking a collaborative approach** — Work with patients from the beginning to help them understand that the behavior is something they do rather than something they are. For therapy to be collaborative, patients should be involved in selecting their own combination of techniques. Plan small but incremental successes, rather than applying a wide range of techniques that overwhelm the patient.

2. **Identifying antecedents to the lapse** — These antecedents can be related to situational, environmental, or cognitive factors. Family history and prior learning can also be associated with the lapse. Often, analyzing the chain of behaviors and cognitions that led to the lapse helps identify points of intervention. Important cognitive antecedents are:

    ▶ Rationalizations utilized

    ▶ Denial of circumstances or feelings

    ▶ Choice points within the chain of events

3. **Using cognitive strategies** — These strategies provide the patient with thought processes regarding change (e.g., "I am changing learned habits rather than personality characteristics," "The change process is a learning process," "Change is a journey."). High-risk situations are similar to dangerous driving conditions in which drivers must exercise extra caution and skill to prevent an accident.

---

**lapse** — mistakes that occur when patients give in to urges with "old" behavior patterns

**relapse** — a total reversal to "old" behavior patterns

**prolapse** — a way of viewing relapses as a slide or fall forward that allows the patient to learn from the relapse

*Since social pressure accounts for 20 percent of relapses, the patients' social interactions may influence them to engage in undesired behaviors. These interactions need to be brought to light and planned for. Many of these situations are considered high risk; however, when effective cognitive or behavioral coping responses can be made, the probability of relapse decreases significantly.[137]*

**relapse rehearsal** — a
technique that uses imagery of
a high-risk situation accompanied by imagery of employing
alternate coping responses

**detachment** — monitoring
urges by observing them come
and go without acting on them

**These strategies include teaching patient to use:**

▶ *Relapse rehearsal*

▶ *Detachment* from their urges, which helps the urges
   to eventually subside.

4. **Incorporating skills training** — Skills training includes
   teaching both cognitive and behavioral responses to
   deal with high-risk situations. This approach includes
   first identifying high-risk situations through monitoring
   ongoing behavior or describing past relapse episodes.
   When patients encounter high-risk situations, they can
   be instructed to "slow down and stop" before proceeding
   any further or to "reconsider the road ahead" or to consult a "road map" for alternate "routes." Then, alternate
   coping strategies can be used.

   **Coping strategies for these high-risk situations
   include problem-solving strategies and conflict
   management.** For those patients whose coping strategies are blocked by fear or anxiety, appropriate anxiety-
   reduction procedures can be used (e.g., relaxation,
   *systematic desensitization*.) General skills training can
   involve direct instruction, modeling, *behavioral rehearsal*,
   coaching, and feedback from the clinician.

**systematic desensitization**
— progressively more
intense exposure to the
feared situation

**behavioral rehearsal** —
during the therapy session,
the clinician helps the patient
rehearse responses to feared
situations

   The knowledge gained from using these skill-building
   exercises gives the patient more choices and better flexibility in responding to future interpersonal situations.

5. **Developing lifestyle interventions** — Building relaxation and exercise into the patient's lifestyle will help
   strengthen the overall coping capacity and reduce the
   stress level of the patient. This can reduce the frequency
   and intensity of the urges toward the old behavior.
   Another form of lifestyle intervention is to teach the
   patient to utilize *substitute indulgences*, or activities to provide the immediate form of self-gratification previously
   experienced by the undesired behavior.

**substitute indulgences** —
alternative indulgences with a
more positive outcome, such
as having a massage, eating
a gourmet meal, exercising,
going to dinner with a friend,
spending leisure time in the
park, or going to a movie

6. **Creating lifestyle balance** — Creating a balance in lifestyle between activities perceived as "shoulds," "have-tos,"
   or "hassles" and those perceived as "pleasurable," "self-ful-
   filling," or "wants." When their lifestyle is weighted down
   with "hassles," patients often associate these hassles with
   a perception of self-deprivation, which leads to a desire
   for indulgence and gratification. Once patients learn to
   recognize and control these contingencies, they should:

   ▶ Set their own standards

   ▶ Monitor their own performance

   ▶ Reinforce themselves appropriately

The relapse prevention treatment example in figure 3.9, below, highlights how the clinician focuses on the maladaptive behavior as "an old habit," taps into the patient's motivation for change, and focuses on the decision-making process. Compare this example with the previous treatment examples; all respond to the same initial comment by the patient.

## Relapse Prevention Efficacy

At this time, there are no controlled outcome studies assessing the effectiveness of using relapse prevention as treatment specifically for BPD.

### Figure 3.9    Relapse Prevention Therapy Treatment Example (Patient = P    Clinician = C)

$P_1$:  **Last time we met I could tell you didn't really care about me, you were just seeing me for the money. I was so mad I went home and cut on my wrists. I couldn't help myself.**

$C_1$:  *You sound pretty angry.*

$P_2$:  You bet I am. I knew you didn't care about me all along.

$C_2$:  *How did feeling angry at me lead you to cut on yourself?*

$P_3$:  Well I was mad at you. I didn't know what to do. I just couldn't stand it anymore.

$C_3$:  *Instead of telling me you were angry with me you went home and hurt yourself. How did you decide to do that?*

$P_4$:  Well I didn't know how mad I was until I left here. Then, I didn't know what to do with my anger, so I did what I'm used to doing.

$C_4$:  *You decided to cut on yourself.*

$P_5$:  Yeah.

$C_5$:  *How did you decide to do that instead of something else?*

$P_6$:  Well, it feels better. Remember, I told you before; it takes the anger away.

$C_6$:  *Remember in the past when you decided you wanted to change that old response pattern? What led you to that decision?*

$P_7$:  Well, it seemed like I just hurt myself and then it didn't really fix things. I'd like to learn how to fix things instead of hurting myself.

$C_7$:  *Next time you are angry with me, let's try to think of something else you could try instead of hurting yourself.*

$P_8$:  Well, when I feel really mad like that I could call you and tell you I'm mad and see if it's true.

$C_8$:  *That's a very good idea. What will you do If I'm not available right then when you call?*

$P_9$:  Well, I can go over to my friend Trudy's house and talk to her. Being with her, I won't cut on myself. If she's not there, I can go walk around the park.

$C_9$:  *I'm glad you have some choices for dealing with that old habit next time. It sounds like feeling angry at me is a high-risk situation for you.*

*The dialog process continues to help the patient identify high-risk situations, connect thoughts and feelings that have led to the old habit in the past, and develop alternate thoughts, feelings, and behaviors for the future.*

# How are Various Individual BPD Therapy Approaches Similar?

Although many differences exist among individual psychotherapy approaches, researchers agree on five basic components as necessary for treating people with BPD:[138]

1. **Creating a stable treatment environment** — Given the capacity of people with BPD to regress into psychotic perceptions, clinicians must clarify and maintain the consistency of roles, schedule, fees, and other boundary issues. Some research indicates that patients perceive this structure as supportive, and it introduces organization into their chaotic lives.[139]

2. **Providing active interventions and responses** — The clinician must be alert and active in identifying, confronting, and directing the patient's behavior, which diminishes transference distortions and provides a framework of clinician supportiveness.

3. **Establishing a connection between the patient's actions and present feelings** — This connection helps patients identify feelings and motives behind their behavior and often includes setting limits on behaviors that threaten the safety of the patient, clinician, or continuation of therapy.

4. **Removing gratification from performing self-destructive behaviors** — The clinician must consistently identify, or help patients identify, the adverse consequences of their self-destructive acts.

5. **Paying careful attention to *countertransference* feelings** — BPD patients have the capacity to evoke feelings of anger and helplessness in the clinician because clinicians perceive them as more dominant and hostile than other patients.[140] Patients can also evoke sustained patterns of countertransference feelings (e.g., the need to be idealized, needed, omnipotent, or submissive). If acted upon, these feelings can be detrimental to the therapeutic relationship and need to be monitored.

Clinicians treating BPD patients should use ongoing supervision to review the patient's progress and to discuss countertransference feelings that may adversely direct the therapy.

**countertransference** —
clinicians' emotions that are triggered by something the patient said or did

# How Can Group Psychotherapy Help Those with BPD?

Many clinicians report that they find group psychotherapy to be the treatment of choice for people with BPD, and many patients value their group therapy experience over individual therapy. A number of clinicians believe individual therapy in conjunction with group therapy is the most effective treatment.[141]

Most theoretical approaches to treating BPD focus on the nature of interpersonal relationships as the cause and the key to maintenance of the disorder. Therefore, group therapy (which offers multiple interpersonal relationships in a controlled setting) gives the person with BPD important opportunities to make the changes necessary for more productive functioning.

*This review focuses on the rationale and benefits for using group therapy conducted by a trained clinician. Specific interventions and techniques are not addressed. The information presented is written for those already experienced in conducting group treatment or those who are planning to refer a patient to group therapy.*

## Treatment Strategies

Group therapy offers a variety of useful approaches that are particularly advantageous for the person with BPD, including:

1. **Reality testing** — Regular feedback from group members is one of the most powerful advantages of group therapy. Patients often accept difficult feedback more easily from peers than from an authority figure (the clinician). The continuous feedback from group members helps decrease interpersonal distortions and intense expressions of primitive fears and needs.

2. **Viewing how the patient relates to others** — Yalom notes that in group therapy, patients will recreate their familial relationships and dynamics (as well as other outside relationships) with members in the group.[125] This provides extremely useful information about the patient's outside relationships for clinicians to use according to their theoretical orientation.

3. **Reducing transference reactions** — These reactions, which are often intense and take a long time to process during individual therapy, are significantly reduced in group therapy. This reduction is due to the increased number of people that provide reality testing and the increased number of recipients of transference reactions.

4. **Healing** — Group therapy offers a healing aspect to people with BPD through the process of being taken seriously and respected by the other group members.

5. **Identification** — During group therapy, people with BPD often watch how the clinician interacts with other group members and internalize some of these behaviors to increase their own coping and interpersonal skills. Additionally, this same *identification* process may take

*Group therapy may be especially helpful for patients who are demanding, egocentric, socially isolated and withdrawn, and socially deviant.[142] Group therapy may be counterproductive when the patient has behavior patterns that are extremely rigid, is antagonistic toward others, is grandiose, and/or harbors a great deal of disdain for others.[141]*

**identification** — process whereby the patient internalizes behavior aspects of important "others"

place with other group members. Hopefully, the patient chooses to identify (internalize) the positive coping skills of other group members rather than the negative ones.

6. **Stimulation** — More schizoid-like (withdrawn) BPD patients may benefit from the stimulation of group interaction.

7. **Peer pressure** — Peer pressure can help set limits for members with poor control over impulsive behaviors.

8. **Changing behavior** — Group therapy provides an avenue for members to be part of a group and to increase their ability to be intimate with others. Group dynamics often center around the methods, including self-mutilation, members use to avoid intimacy. Group therapy is an avenue for changing these patterns.

### Group Psychotherapy Efficacy

Several controlled studies have been done assessing the effectiveness of group therapy for people with BPD.[93, 111, 142–144] The results of these studies indicate decreases in parasuicidal behavior, improved work status, and improvement in severe BPD symptoms. Research conducted on Yalom's curative factors indicates that the most helpful group factors for people with BPD are *universality* and *existential factors*.[141, 145]

**universality** — the sense of not being alone in one's struggles

**existential factors** — social aloneness, self-responsibility, coming to terms with mortality

# How Can Psychological Treatment Strategies be used to Manage Suicide Risk?

Once a clinician has determined that a patient is suicidal, the first key treatment issue is whether or not the patient should be hospitalized. After making a decision to hospitalize, the clinician needs to ensure that the person evaluating the crisis has sufficient evidence for making such a decision. For example, a patient who is angry or does not want to be hospitalized may convince police officers or mental health workers (depending on state law) that there is a misunderstanding, and they do not want to kill themselves. This could result in a suicidal patient being released.

*One of the most widely cited works on standards of care for suicidal patients is Bruce Bongar's classic work, **The Suicidal Patient**.[146]*

The clinician then reduces the ongoing potential for suicide after the initial suicidal crisis by:[89]

- ▶ Including the family in treatment
- ▶ Realistically informing the patient about probable treatment length and effectiveness as well as his/her expected role

▶ Regularly questioning the patient about suicidal feelings, intent, and plans (including possible repeated use of a suicide risk instrument)

The clinician should ensure that any "gatekeeping" evaluator understands the patient's history, suicidal symptoms and plans, and the risk factors that led to the referral. In addition, the clinician should be sure that the hospital can provide the level of restraint necessary to ensure the patient's safety. In most cases, the clinician will be expected to provide hospital staff with specific patient information identifying the need for inpatient hospital care after intake. Additionally, the clinician needs to maintain contact with the hospital treating staff about discharge planning for the patient.

*The clinician may be able to contact a family member or friend to have guns (or medications) taken away/locked up. In this case, the suicidal individual will not necessarily find another method.[147]*

Once the patient is discharged, the clinician can develop an outpatient treatment plan, featuring:

▶ An explicit plan for future suicidal crises, which includes: regular reviews of suicidal ideation, intent, plan, and status of risk factors as well as patient and family involvement

▶ Increased session frequency and/or scheduled, between-visit contacts (e.g., via phone)

▶ Steps for removing potential suicide instruments, perhaps with help from family or friends

▶ Regular evaluation of the patient's willingness to emotionally engage in the treatment relationship and responsiveness to treatment

▶ (For the clinician), professional consultations (and documented results) with a colleague experienced in patient management

## Using Suicide Contracts

A common suicide intervention for clinicians, prior to hospitalization, is to specifically contract with the patient to not commit suicide. This is a fairly common procedure when clinicians believe the risk may be minimal or chronic in nature. Contracts are usually a verbal or written agreement between the clinician and patient that the person will not commit suicide without using the emergency plan developed or without first speaking with the clinician.

*Although the use of so-called "no-harm contracts" is controversial, overall, many studies find that most individuals, both professionals and lay persons, are positive about the use of such agreements.[90, 91]*

Use these contracts with caution because:

▶ Some patients think the contract means that they should contact their clinician only when they are acutely suicidal and desperate.

*As a clinical (rather than legal) tool, these contracts may provide information about the patient's level of suicidal intent and their sense of control.*

*Some contracts add a basic promise to call a crisis line if the patient stops taking medications, seriously thinks about committing suicide, or takes any action towards planning suicide.[87]*

*These strategies are consistent with a recent study pointing out that, while there is a need for more research on treatment effectiveness for suicidal patients, cognitive-behavioral approaches that emphasize a problem-solving focus seem to reduce suicidal behavior for most persons studied, at least for short-term interventions.[92] The data from multiple attempters in this study suggests that longer-term treatment may be needed to address underlying personality disorders and to develop personal skills for accessing resources and coping with life crises.*

▶ Others may have a strong need to be compliant and reasonable and may sign a contract despite serious misgivings about living up to it — precipitating a crisis due to feelings of guilt and shame.

▶ Clinicians might gain a false sense of security from such a contract.

More explicit contracts appear more useful than general contracts with suicidal patients because they promote patients:[91]

▶ Agreeing with specific therapeutic treatment goals, including to "live a long life with more pleasure and less unhappiness than I have now"

▶ Learning better ways to manage their emotions

▶ Specifically naming contact and backup persons with phone numbers

▶ Working with their clinician

▶ "Openly renegotiating" the contract when it expires

In contrast, general contracts require the patient to sign a statement that, for a specific time, they would speak with a friend or relative if feeling suicidal.

## Using Psychotherapy for Suicidal Patients

Until the crisis is over and the patient is no longer intensely suicidal, psychotherapy should focus on increasing the patient's sense of choices available to them and their sense of being emotionally supported. Key strategies include:

▶ Reducing psychiatric symptom intensity (e.g., instilling a sense of hope, decreasing vegetative symptoms, teaching methods to cope with anxiety and frustration, etc.)

▶ Teaching problem-solving methods to cope with major life stressors, such as divorce or unemployment

For first-time attempters, once the immediate suicidal crisis is past, the best way to reduce potential attempts is to immediately try to reduce the symptoms or mitigate the life event producing the crisis. For multiple attempters, this strategy's value may be limited. More intensive follow-up of longer duration should focus on reducing what precipitated the immediate crisis and on achieving longer-term ability to prevent future crises.[148]

Involving family members or other concerned parties in evaluating and responding to suicide risk can be advantageous.[149] They typically provide increased social support for the distressed patient, valuable information for evaluating ongoing risk, and backup safety options should the suicide risk increase between clinical contacts.

## Understanding Key Issues Impacting Suicide Treatment Strategies

Treating suicidal patients often involves dealing with issues outside those of typical treatment environments, including:

▶ **Dealing with insurance restrictions/limitations** — Managed care and similar organizations may restrict patient care even during a suicidal crisis. Although this situation is being slowly addressed via court cases (e.g., Andrews-Clarke v. Travelers), clinicians may need to talk with patients about coverage restrictions and advocate on a patient's behalf to appeal these decisions.[150]

*Hospital choice also may hinge on whether or not the patient has insurance. Once hospitalized (whether voluntarily or not), clinicians should be involved in the facility's ongoing treatment and discharge planning.*

Clinicians need to become familiar with state laws and procedures for involuntarily committing a suicidal patient to a facility, considering the patient's insurance benefits and the willingness to be voluntarily hospitalized.

▶ **Using confidentiality waivers** — Suicidal patients need to know that confidentiality may be waived to protect their safety and that the clinician will take their suicidal thoughts and comments seriously. Clinicians who wish to know more about the potential legal ramifications of a specific waiver should consult an attorney.

▶ **Developing an emergency plan** — Develop an emergency plan for outpatients who display suicidal or even homicidal behaviors. Discuss this plan with the patient early in the first session, providing a written procedure to follow in an emergency.

*Although emergency plans vary widely, they often include calling 911, contacting the clinician after hours through a phone service or on-call line, or making use of community-based crisis hotlines.*

▶ **Recognizing countertransference issues** — These issues often occurs when the clinician reacts to the patient with their own sense of helplessness, worries about being able to handle a suicidal crisis, and fear of potential legal outcomes. This reaction is magnified by the suicidal person's negative experiences of telling others about their thoughts, making them leery of sharing this information with the clinician because they expect the same reaction. Clinicians who present themselves as competent, calm, and able to take action may help resolve the crisis and calm the patient.

▶ **Handling legal concerns** — To mitigate the risk of liability, clinicians should focus on the patient's health and well-being, following prudent standards for decision making and documentation, such as:

*In malpractice or negligence cases, courts and juries tend to evaluate the situation in terms of how "reasonable" the clinician's actions were in comparison to those of "average," prudent clinicians of similar training and experience.[146] Courts do not expect clinicians to have perfect judgment and accept that predicting suicide can be an almost impossible task.[146, 151]*

  ▶ Documenting specific findings on the patient's degree of risk, the clinician's reasoning during the crisis, and decisions made

  ▶ Consulting with other professionals and documenting these consultations, particularly when managing a suicidal patient on an outpatient basis

## Key Concepts for Chapter Three

1. Key environmental influences that appear to be linked to BPD are history of physical/sexual abuse and having witnessed serious domestic violence.

2. Individual psychotherapeutic approaches to treating BPD include psychodynamic, psychoanalytic, interpersonal, cognitive, dialectical behavior, cognitive analytic, and relapse prevention.

3. Psychodynamic therapy helps those with BPD identify their feelings and how those feelings reflect a reaction to past events, remedying intrapsychic conflicts.

4. Psychoanalytic therapy uses maintenance of neutrality and interpretation to help the patient identify and cope with aggressive feelings rather than repress them.

5. Interpersonal psychotherapy focuses on identifying and altering maladaptive communication styles and behaviors.

6. Cognitive therapy addresses the unrealistic expectations those with BPD have about current relationships based on cognitions developed early in life.

7. Dialectical behavior (DBT) theorists focus on often-opposing forces that produce the dysfunction characteristic of BPD, especially suicidal behavior.

8. DBT has proven more effective for treating BPD than treatment as usual in the community and than medication therapy alone.

9. Relapse prevention focuses on teaching the patient to change addictive behaviors and create a more balanced lifestyle.

10. Group therapy is especially valuable for patients who are demanding, egocentric, socially isolated/withdrawn, or socially deviant.

11. Inpatient care issues for suicidal patients involve clear communication between clinician and hospital, oversight of discharge planning, and development of an explicit plan for preventing future suicide crisis once the patient has been discharged from the hospital.

12. Outpatient care typically involves use of a suicide contract that the patient signs, agreeing to talk to someone when feeling suicidal.

# Chapter Four:
# Biological Approaches to Treating BPD

*This chapter answers the following:*

---

▶ **What are the Genetic Indications for BPD?** — This section presents research on genetic and environmental factors that may be linked to BPD.

▶ **What are the Neurological Indications for BPD?** — This section discusses symptom clusters related to neurochemical systems in the brain as well as neurobiological abnormalities in those with BPD.

▶ **What Medications are used to Treat BPD, and How Effective are They?** — This section presents the medications currently used to treat BPD, including side effects and efficacy.

S OME research indicates that BPD may be of a genetic, neurological, and/or biological origin. Theoretical approaches based on this research promote the use of *psychopharmacological* treatments for those with BPD. This review focuses on genetic as well as neurological and/ or biological indications of BPD and addresses medication treatment strategies and efficacy.

**psychopharmacological** — medications that affect thought processes, mood, and behavior

## What are the Genetic Indications for BPD?

Research indicates that BPD is about five times more common among first-degree, biological relatives of those with the disorder than those in the general population.[8] This finding could either be due to genetic links or could indicate the impact of environmental influences on the disorder. Further genetic information comes from research conducted in the 1980s that found parents of those with BPD to have a low incidence of schizophrenia and a high incidence of affective disorder.[152]

Also during the 1980s, researchers found that biological markers of sleep latency and "Rapid Eye Movement" (REM) measurements were similar among those with BPD and those with major depressive disorder. However, these findings have subsequently been refuted, and new auditory biological markers (auditory 300) now link BPD more closely to schizophrenia.[154]

# What are the Neurobiological Indications for BPD?

Throughout BPD literature, four prominent clusters of BPD symptoms emerge with different underlying neurochemical systems:[155–158]

1. **Affective instability** — This cluster of symptoms is related to abnormalities in the brain's *adrenergic* and *cholinergic* systems.

   Symptoms include labile affect, irritability including inappropriate and intense outbursts of anger, mood instability, low mood or dysphoria, and stress-related *decompensation*.[159]

2. **Depression** — This cluster of symptoms is related to abnormalities in the brain's adrenergic and cholinergic systems.

   Symptoms include depressed mood, loss of interest in life's activities and pleasures, insomnia or hypersomnia, poor attention and concentration, and recurrent suicidal ideation.

3. **Transient psychoticism** — Abnormalities in central *dopaminergic* systems may underlie transient psychotic experiences. The *neurotransmitter* dopamine appears to be important in motor control systems, *limbic* systems, and schizophrenia.

   Symptoms of transient, stress-related psychoticism include referential thinking, derealization or depersonalization, paranoia, distortion of reality, and magical thinking.

4. **Impulsive aggressive behavior** — Abnormalities in central nervous system serotonergic functioning appear to underlie impulsive aggressive behaviors, particularly suicide attempts.[157–165] The central *serotonergic* neurotransmitter system — 5-HT — appears to be one component modulating aggression and impulsivity. Research with patients who have BPD indicates that:

   ▶ They have lower 5-HT1A receptor sensitivity, affecting impulsive aggression and suicidality.[166, 167]

   ▶ Those who suffered severe traumatic stress in childhood had blunted response to a serotonergic agonist — M-CPP.[166]

   ▶ High levels of the cerebrospinal fluid concentration of monoamine metabolites 5-hydoxyindoleacetic acid (5-HIAA) appear to protect against impulsive or suicidal behavior.[163]

   Symptoms include suicidal and parasuicidal behavior, self-mutilation, food or alcohol binges, promiscuity, assaultive behavior, and antisocial acts.

**adrenergic** — a neuronal pathway in the adrenal gland that produces adrenaline (also known as epinephrine)

**cholinergic** — neurons and neural pathways that release the neurotransmitter, acetylcholine, which is involved in stimulating sweat glands and fibers to skeletal muscles

**decompensation** — a failure of one's defense mechanisms leading to an exacerbation of BPD symptoms

**dopaminergic** — neural pathways in which the neurotransmitter dopamine (which appears to inhibit motor control systems and limbic activity) is involved

**neurotransmitter** — chemical agents that affect behavior, mood, and feelings

**limbic** — associated with autonomic functions and certain aspects of emotions and behavior

**serotonergic** — neurons and neural pathways that release the neurotransmitter serotonin

## Neurobiological Abnormalities

Further support for a biological component to BPD comes from research indicating brain abnormalities in those with BPD. Specifically, 40 percent of BPD subjects showed non-localized brain dysfunction in the form of abnormally diffuse, slow activity, noted from recorded electroencephalograms (EEGs).[168] Some research indicates a pattern of low volume in these brain regions:[169]

1. **Hippocampus** (plays a part in memory, navigation)

2. **Amygdala** (regulates mood, emotion)

3. **Orbito frontal** and **dorsolateral prefrontal cortex** (regulate many complex brain functions including memory, perceptual awareness, "thinking," language, and consciousness)

4. **Anterior cingulated cortex** (also plays a part in memory)

Some researchers theorize that those with BPD suffer from a hyperarousal dyscontrol syndrome involving limbic and pre-frontal circuits.[170] These studies found somewhat mixed results, such as:

▶ When presented with emotional facial expressions, those with BPD (vs. controls) showed significantly greater activation of the left amygdala.[171]

▶ Those with BPD (vs. controls) in another study showed no physiological sign of hyper-responsiveness to emotional expression (via measures of heart rate, skin conductance, and startle response).[172]

▶ Full frontal lobe maturation was unsuccessful in patients with BPD as measured by event-related brain potentials.[173]

## From the Patient's Perspective

*I know I am feeling a lot better lately but Owen thinks that medications may help me still more. She is happy that I am not cutting on myself as much when I get upset and don't feel as afraid that Alex is going to leave me. She says the medication may help me feel even more stable. I guess I'll give them a try; they might help me not feel so afraid, anxious, and upset.*

**visiospatial** — environmental
spatial relationships that are
processed visually

Cognitive mechanisms also appear to be involved in BPD. Some research suggests biological differences between patients with BPD and others of impaired *visiospatial* processing that requires learning and recall of novel, complex information. Additional deficits appear in visiospatial discrimination, speed, and fluency. These findings do not appear to be related to depression, psychomotor deficits, or attention problems. Additionally, Rorschach studies have found deviant communication patterns, an inability to maintain or shift cognitive sets, and odd reasoning.[161] These results suggest patchy, underdeveloped cognitive functioning among those with BPD that is, at this point, still of uncertain origin.

Despite indications of abnormal limbic and prefrontal cortex functioning, there is little evidence of cognitive performance deficits. One study found those with BPD had slower perceptual speed and slower working memory than controls with deficits not augmented by increased cognitive demands.[34] Other studies found no differences between those with BPD and controls on cognitive executive functioning tasks, such as planning, problem solving, or memory.[174, 175]

# What Medications are used to Treat BPD, and How Effective are They?

Prescribing medication can:

► *Reduce the motivation for psychotherappy*

► *Be perceived as a negative indicator of the patient's condition*

► *Increase cognitive functioning, which can enhance psychotherapy*

Although there are numerous psychopharmacological interventions for BPD, researchers have found no single medication superior to another for the disorder's broad-spectrum symptoms.[176–178] Deciding which psychopharmacological agent to prescribe depends on the presenting symptoms.[157, 158, 176]

Medications appear to mostly address three primary symptom clusters: impulsive/aggressive behavioral dyscontrol, affective instability, and cognitive/perceptual disturbances.[156, 157, 179, 180]

*Due to the suicide potential of those with BPD, the prescribing physician must carefully consider medication lethality and the number of pills given in a single prescription.*

There are relatively few placebo-controlled, double-blind outcome studies for BPD treatment. Those medications with positive controlled outcome data include (shown in bold in figure 4.1):

► **Divalproex sodium** for irritability, anger, and impulsive aggression[181, 182]

► **Fluvoxamine** for affective instability (rapid mood shifts)[183]

► **Olanzapine** for all three symptom groups (affective, cognitive/perceptual, impulsive/aggressive)[184–186]

► **Topiramate** for anger[187]

► **E-EPA (omega 3 fatty acid)** for aggressive and depressive symptoms[188]

Clinicians have found medication treatment most effective for acute symptoms, with limited efficacy when used for maintenance.[157, 158, 176] Medication types used to treat BPD symptoms include:

- ▶ Selective Serotonin Reuptake Inhibitors (SSRIs)
- ▶ Selective Serotonin Norepinephrine Reuptake Inhibitors (SSNRIs)
- ▶ A Norepinephrine Reuptake Inhibitor (NRI)
- ▶ Antipsychotic Medications (Atypical and Typical)
- ▶ Anticonvulsants
- ▶ An Opiate Antagonist
- ▶ An Antimanic Agent
- ▶ Benzodiazepines
- ▶ An Omega 3 Fatty Acid
- ▶ An Antihypertensive Agent

*Figure 4.1 (on pages 62 through 63) lists these medications in terms of medication class and name, target symptoms affected, and common side effects.*

## Figure 4.1    Medications Used to Treat BPD Target Symptoms

| Medication Class / • Name | Target Symptoms | Common Side Effects |
|---|---|---|
| SSRIs<br>• Citalopram<br>• Fluoxetine<br>• **Fluvoxamine**[183, 189]<br>• Paroxetine<br>• Sertraline | impulsive/aggressive<br>affective instability<br>depression | Sexual dysfunction, decreased appetite, nausea, fatigue, daytime sedation, nervousness, restlessness, anxiety, agitation, respiratory complaints, headache, dry mouth, tremors, diarrhea or constipation, insomnia, anorexia or increased weight gain, frequent urination, dizziness, and sweating.<br><br>**Except for fluoxetine,** rapid discontinuation of SSRIs is commonly associated with symptoms of withdrawal, which persist for 1–2 weeks. Typical SSRI withdrawal symptoms include dizziness, headache, tingling, "electric-shock" sensations, and flu-like symptoms. |
| SSNRIs<br>• Duloxetine<br>• Venlafaxine | affective instability | **For duloxetine:** Appetite changes, constipation, diarrhea, dizziness, dry mouth, fatigue, headache, insomnia, nausea, sexual difficulties, sleepiness, sweating, tremor, urinary difficulties, vomiting, weakness.<br><br>**For venlafaxine:** Abnormal ejaculation/orgasm, anxiety, blurred vision, constipation, dizziness, dry mouth, impotence, insomnia, nausea, nervousness, sleepiness, sweating, tremor, vomiting, weakness, weight loss. |
| NRI<br>• Bupropion | affective instability | Dry mouth and sleeplessness. |
| Atypical Antipsychotics<br>• Aripiprazole<br>• Clozapine[190, 191]<br>• **Olanzapine**[184-186]<br>• Quetiapine<br>• Risperidone[192]<br>• Ziprasidone<br><br>Typical Antipsychotics<br>• Chlorpromazine<br>• Haloperidol<br>• Molindone<br>• Perphanazine<br>• Thioridazine | impulsive/aggressive<br>affective instability<br>depression | Blurred vision, urinary retention, dry mouth, constipation, decreased sweating, and memory difficulty.<br><br>Less common side effects are acute dyskinesia (muscle spasms), akathisia (extreme restlessness), Parkinsonism (tremor, very flat affect, poor sensory-motor coordination, exhaustion, and loss of ability to initiate action), neuroleptic malignant syndrome (hyperthermia, muscle rigidity, flushing, unstable blood pressure, tachycardia), and tardive dyskinesia (irreversible Parkinsonism). |

**Note**: Medications shown in bold type are those for which positive controlled outcome data currently exists.

## Figure 4.1 continued

| Medication Class / • Name | Target Symptoms | Common Side Effects |
|---|---|---|
| Anticonvulsants<br>• Carbamazepine<br>• **Divalproex** (valproic acid)[181, 182, 193]<br>• Lamotrigine[194]<br>• Oxcarbazepine<br>• **Topiramate**[187] | impulsive/aggressive<br>affective instability | Itching, hives, rashes, hypotension, hypertension, congestive heart failure, urinary retention, dizziness, fatigue, incoordination, visual disturbance, speech disturbance, depression, and gastrointestinal distress. This drug may cause lethal bone marrow suppression and thus must be used with complete blood count monitoring (CBC).<br><br>**For carbamazepine and topiramate:** Note that both medications decrease the effectiveness of estradiol birth control pills.<br><br>**For valproic acid and divalproex:** Pancreatitis is rare but serious and occurs early in treatment. Hepatitis most common in children, usually within first 6 months of treatment. |
| Opiate Antagonist<br>• Naltrexone[195] | impulsive/aggressive<br>affective instability<br>cognitive/peripheral disturbances | Nausea, insomnia, headache, anxiety, fatigue, dizziness, weight loss, and joint and muscle pain. |
| Antimanic Agent<br>• Lithium carbonate | impulsive/aggressive<br>cognitive/peripheral disturbances | Nausea, cramps, diarrhea, hand tremor, muscle weakness, fatigue, insomnia, thirst, headache, and decreased concentration. Less common side effects include weight gain, hypothyroidism, polydipsia (drinking of extreme amounts of water), and skin rashes. |
| Benzodiazepines<br>• Clonazepam<br>• Diazepam<br>• Lorazepam | cognitive/peripheral disturbances; contraindicated for impulsive/aggressive due to increase in behavioral dyscontrol, including suicide attempts and other behavioral outbursts | Drowsiness, light-headedness, fatigue, weakness, loss of coordination. Less common side effects include confusion, hallucinations, depression, amnesia, paradoxical stimulation of hyperactivity, insomnia, rage, and anxiety. |
| Omega 3 Fatty Acid<br>• **E-EPA (Ethyl-eicosapentaenoic acid)**[188] | aggression<br>depression | Mild gastrointestinal upset; halitosis; eructation; "fishy-smelling" breath, skin, urine; occasional nosebleeds; easy bruising. **Note:** Use with caution for those taking blood-thinning medications or those with hemophelia. |
| Antihypertensive Agent<br>• Clonidine[196] | acute states of impulsive/aggressive (average inner tension and urge to commit self-injurious behavior)<br>cognitive/perceptual (dissociative) | Hypotension, sedation, dizziness, fatigue, dry mouth, nausea, constipation, sexual dysfunction, insomnia, anxiety, depression, weight gain, sensitivity to light, and rash. |

**Note**: Medications shown in bold type are those for which positive controlled outcome data currently exists.

## Key Concepts for Chapter Four

**1.** Those with BPD suffer symptoms arising from abnormalities in the brain's adrenergic, cholinergic, dopiminergic, and serotonergic systems.

**2.** Neurobiological abnormalities associated with BPD appear in the hippocampus, amygdala, orbito frontal and dorso lateral prefrontal cortex as well as the anterior cingulated cortex.

**3.** A key benefit of combining medications with psychotherapy for those with BPD is the medication's tendency to improve central nervous system functioning, thereby making many patients more cognitively and verbally accessible to psychotherapy.

**4.** Medications used to treat BPD differ in the target symptoms for which they are most effective and tend to be more appropriate for treating acute symptoms rather than for maintenance.

**5.** Medication classes used for treating BPD include SSRIs, SSNRIs, antipsychotics, anticonvulsants, and benzodiazepines as well as an NRI, opiate antagonist, antimanic agent, antihypertensive, and an omega 3 fatty acid.

# Glossary

## A

**active passivity** — the tendency to approach problems in a passive and helpless manner

**adrenergic** — a neuronal pathway in the adrenal gland that produces adrenaline (also known as epinephrine)

**affect** — emotion; feeling; mood

**apparent competency syndrome** — the tendency to appear deceptively competent

## B

**behavioral rehearsal** — during the therapy session, the clinician helps the patient rehearse responses to feared situations

**balanced lifestyle** — a lifestyle in which the patient has control of their behavior and chooses generally moderate behaviors

**bereavement overload** — overwhelming number of feelings related to grief and loss

**blocking** — disruption or inhibition of thought processes

## C

**clarification** — exploration of vague or contradictory data

**cholinergic** — neurons and neural pathways that release the neurotransmitter, acetylcholine, which is involved in stimulating sweat glands and fibers to skeletal muscles

**collaborative** — clinician and patient putting equal effort toward agreed-upon goals

**compulsive** — feeling compelled to act against one's wishes

**confrontation** — drawing the patients' attention to data that is discrepant or outside of their awareness

**contingency** — an agreement between the clinician and patient regarding specific behaviors that will be followed by specific reinforcers or punishers

**convergent validity** — when test results positively correlate with other instruments measuring the same variable

**countertransference** — clinicians' emotions that are triggered by something the patient said or did

# D

**decompensation** — a failure of one's defense mechanisms leading to an exacerbation of BPD symptoms

**delusions** — beliefs maintained despite much evidence or argument to the contrary

**denial** — the process whereby the patient responds to an event as if it is not or has not happened

**depersonalization** — a sense that one has lost contact with one's own personal reality (e.g., "My body feels strange, like it's not my own.")

**derealization** — a sense that one has lost contact with external reality

**detachment** — monitoring urges by observing them come and go without acting on them

**devaluation** — the process whereby the client undervalues the abilities and/or intentions of others

**dialectical** — systematic reasoning processes where a person tries to resolve contradictory ideas

**dichotomous thinking** — tendency to perceive and characterize situations, others' actions, and solutions as "black or white," "all or nothing," "good or bad," "trustworthy or deceitful," "successful or complete failures"

**discriminant validity** — an instrument's ability to discriminate BPD from other disorders

**dissociation** — an abnormal psychological state in which one's perception of oneself and/or one's environment is altered significantly

**dissociative ego states** — attitudes and emotions that produce anxiety become separated from the rest of the person's personality and function independently

**dopaminergic** — neural pathways in which the neurotransmitter dopamine (which appears to inhibit motor control systems and limbic activity) is involved

**dysphoric** — generalized feeling of distress

# E

**electroconvulsive therapy (ECT)** — a type of treatment that induces a seizure through an external electrical source often used to treat depression

**emotional dysregulation** — emotional imbalance or poor emotional control

**eurosis** — non-physiological disorder characterized by high levels of anxiety but no impairment in reality testing

**existential factors** — social aloneness, self-responsibility, coming to terms with mortality

# H

**hallucinations** — hearing or seeing things others do not

**hyperphrasia** — pathologically excessive talking

# I

**idealization** — the process whereby the client sees another person as only "good" or "perfect" frustrating to others

**identification** — process whereby the patient internalizes behavior aspects of important "others"

**impulsive** — acting without first thinking about the action

**interpretation** — verbally giving meaning to the link between the patient's unmet needs and current actions

**interrater reliability** — degree that different raters agree on a diagnosis based on the use of the instrument

**intrapsychic** — psychological processes within a person

# L

**labile affect** — marked and rapid mood shifts

**lapse** — mistakes that occur when patients give in to urges with "old" behavior patterns

**limbic** — associated with autonomic functions and certain aspects of emotions and behavior

# M

**maladaptive behavior patterns** — patterns of behavior likely to produce so much psychic distress that therapy is necessary

**micropsychotic symptoms** — minor psychotic symptoms

**mild formal thought disorder** — disturbances in speech, communication, and/or thinking

**mistakes** — recurrences of behaviors being "unlearned" and framed as mistakes to be learned from

# N

**neurotransmitter** — chemical agents that affect behavior, mood, and feelings

# O

**object relations** — present or past relationships with these love "objects" — "others" who are the focus of love or affection

# P

**paranoia** — having suspicions and beliefs that one is being followed, plotted against, persecuted, etc.

**pathological internalized object relations** — extremely dysfunctional relationships with the love objects, which are now carried by the patient as internal beliefs about relationships in general

**projective identification** — the process whereby the patient behaves toward others in such a manner that elicits the very behavior that will confirm their own underlying beliefs

**projective measure of personality (as measured by the Rorschach)** — the stimuli or inkblots are assumed to be neutral, created randomly with no specific shape nor function; patient perceptions of shapes, movement, and other elements seen as products of their own experiences and perceptual orientation projected on the cards

**prolapse** — a way of viewing relapses as a slide or fall forward that allows the patient to learn from the relapse

**psychic deficit** — inadequately developed sense of self

**psychopharmacological** — medications that affect thought processes, mood, and behavior

**psychosis** — grossly impaired reality testing

**psychotic depression** — severe depression that includes delusions (false beliefs) or hallucinations (perceptual distortions)

**psychotic transference** — grossly impaired reality testing regarding transference issues

**psychotropic medications** — medications that affect behavior, emotions, and/or cognitive processes

# R

**reciprocal roles** — thoughts and actions directed toward eliciting or predicting a particular response

**referential thinking** — mistakenly believing others' actions or external events are specifically related to one's self

**regression** — reverting or retreating into an earlier, more childlike pattern of behavior

**relapse** — a total reversal to "old" behavior patterns

**relapse rehearsal** — a technique that uses imagery of a high-risk situation accompanied by imagery of employing alternate coping responses

# S

**schemas** — organized belief systems that attach meaning to events

**sensitivity ratio** — cases correctly diagnosed

**serotonergic** — neurons and neural pathways that release the neurotransmitter serotonin

**specificity ratio** — non-cases correctly identified

**splitting** — the division of self and others into "all good" or "all bad" categories, which results in sudden reversals of feelings and conceptualizations about one's self and others

**substitute indulgences** — alternative indulgences with a more positive outcome, such as having a massage, eating a gourmet meal, exercising, going to dinner with a friend, spending leisure time in the park, or going to a movie

**systematic desensitization** — progressively more intense exposure to the feared situation

## T

**taxonomy** — classification system

**transference** — patients respond to clinicians based on particular images of themselves, particular images or beliefs about clinicians, and emotional reactions that connect the two

## U

**universality** — the sense of not being alone in one's struggles

**unrelenting crisis** — the individual does not return to an emotional baseline before the next crisis hits

## V

**validity** — degree that the instrument measures what it purports to measure

**visiospatial** — environmental spatial relationships that are processed visually

## W

**wise mind** — the part of the person that pays attention and attaches meaning to all that is happening around them.

# References

1. Paris, J. (2004). Borderline or bipolar? Distinguishing borderline personality disorder from bipolar spectrum disorders. *Harvard Review of Psychiatry, 12(3),* 140-5.

2. Smith, D.J., Muir, W.J., Blackwood, D.H. (2004). Is borderline personality disorder part of the bipolar spectrum? *Harvard Review of Psychiatry, 12(3),* 133-9.

3. Magill, C.A. (2004). The boundary between borderline personality disorder and bipolar disorder: Current concepts and challenges. *Canadian Journal of Psychiatry, 49(8),* 551-6.

4. Deltito, J., Martin, L., Riefkohl, J., Austria, B., Kissilenko, A., Corless, C., Morse, P. (2001). Do patients with borderline personality disorder belong to the bipolar spectrum? *Journal of Affective Disorders, 67(1-3),* 221-8.

5. Kroll, Carey, Sines, and Rothe. (1982). Are there borderlines in Britain? A cross-validation of U.S. findings. *Archives of General Psychiatry, 39,* 60-63.

6. Ronningstam, E. & Gunderson, J. (1991) . Differentiating borderline personality disorder from narcissistic personality disorder. *Journal of Personality Disorders, 5(3),* 225-232.

7. Gross, R., Olfson, M., Gameroff, M., Shea, S., Feder, A., Fuentes, M., Lantigua, R., Weissman, M.M. (2002) Borderline personality disorder in primary care. *Archives of Internal Medicine, 162(1),* 53-60.

8. American Psychiatric Association. (2000) . *Diagnostic and statistical manual of mental disorders. (4th ed.), Text Revision,* Washington, D.C.: American Psychiatric Association.

9. American Psychiatric Association. (1987). *Diagnostic and statistical manual of mental disorders (3rd ed., rev. ed.).* Washington, DC: Author.

10. Swartz, M., Blazer, D., George, L, & Winfield, I. (1990). Estimating the prevalence of borderline personality disorder in the community. *Journal of Personality Disorders, 4(3),* 257-272.

11. Bellack, A.S., & Hersen, M. (1990). *Handbook of comparative treatment for adult disorders.* New York: John Wiley & Sons.

12. Stone, M.H., Hurt, S. W., & Stone, K. (1987). Long-term follow-up of borderline inpatients meeting DSM-III criteria: I. Global outcome. *Journal of Personality Disorders, 1(4),* 291-298.

13. Trull, T.J., Useda, J.D., Conforti, K., & Doan, B.T. (1997). Borderline personality disorder features in nonclinical young adults: Two-year outcome. *Journal of Abnormal Psychology, 106(2),* 307-314.

14. Links, P.S., Helelgrave, R., & van Reekum, R. (1999). Impulsivity: Core aspect of borderline personality disorder. *Journal of Personality Disorders, 13(1),* 1-9.

15. Paris, Joel (1990). Completed suicide in borderline personality disorder. *Psychiatric Annals, 20(1),* 19-21.

16. Paris, J. (2002). Implications of long-term outcome research for the management of patients with borderline personality disorder. *Harvard Review of Psychiatry, 10(6),* 315-23.

17. Zanarini, M.C., Frankenburg, F.R., Hennen, J., Silk, K.R. (2003). The longitudinal course of borderline psychopathology; 6-year prospective follow-up of the phenmenology of borderline personality disorder. *American Journal of Psychiatry, 160(2),* 274-83.

18. Zanarini, M.C., Frankenburg, F.R., Hennen, J., Silk, K.R. (2004) Mental health service utilization by borderline personality disorder patients and Axis II comparison subjects followed prospectively for 6 years. *Journal of Clinical Psychology, 65(1),* 28-36.

19. Stevenson, J., Meares, R., Comerford, A., (2003). Diminished impulsivity in older patients with borderline personality disorder. *American Journal of Psychiatry, 160(1),* 165-6.

20. Stone, M., Hurt, S. W., & Stone (1987). The PI 500: Long-term follow-up of borderline inpatients meeting DSM-III criteria. I. Global outcome. *Journal of Personality Disorders, 1(4),* 291-298.

21. Skodol, A.E., Gunderson, J.G., McGlashan, T.H., Dyck, I.R., Stout, R.L., Bender, D.S., Grilo, C.M., Shea, M.T., Zanarini, M.C., Morey, L.C., Sanislow, C.A., Oldham, J.M. (2002). Functional impairment in patients with schizotypal, borderline, avoidant, or obsessive-compulsive personality disorder. *American Journal of Psychiatry, 159(2),* 276-83.

22. Siegel, M.A. , Landes, A., Foster, C.D. (Eds.) (1993). *Health — A concern for every American.* Wylie, TX: Information Plus.

23. Solof, P.H. Lynch, K.G., Kelly, T.M., Malone, K.M. & Mann, J.J. (2000). Characteristics of suicide attempts of patients with major depressive episode and borderline personality disorder: A comparative study. *American Journal of Psychiatry, 157,* 601-608.

24. Plakun, E. M. (1991). Prediciton of outcome in borderline personality disorder. *Journal of Personality Disorders, 5(2),* 93-101.

25. Paris, J., Brown, R. & Nowlis, D. (1987). Long-term follow-up of borderline patients in a general hospital. *Comprehensive Psychiatry, 28,* 530-535.

26. Tidemalm, D., Elofsson, S., Stefansson, C.G., Waern, M., Runeson, B. (2005). Predictors of suicide in a community-based cohort of individuals with severe mental disorder. *Soc Psychiatry Psychiatr Epidemiol 40(8)*:595-600.

27. Zanarini, M.C.; Frankenburg, F.R. Hermen, J., Reich, D.B., Silk, K.R. (2004) Axis 1 cormobidity in patients with borderline personality disorder: 6-year follow-up and prediction of time to remission. *American Journal of Psychiatry, 161(11),* 2108-14.

28. Zanarini, M. C., Gunderson, J. G., Frankenburg, F. R., Chauncey, D. L., & Glutting, J. H. (1991). The face validity of the DSM-III and DSM-III-R criteria sets for borderline personality disorder. *American Journal of Psychiatry, 148(7),* 870-874.

29. Sanislow, C.A., Grilo, C.M., Morey, L.C., Bemder, D.S., Skodol, A.E., Gunderson, J.G., Shea, M.T., Stout, R.L., Zanarini, M.C., McGlashan, T.H. (2002). Confirmatory factor analysis of DSM-IV criteria for borderline personality disorder: Findings from the collaborative longitudinal personality disorders study. *American Journal of Psychiatry, 159(2),* 284-90.

30. Blais, M.S., Hilsenroth, M.J., & Fowler, J.C. (1999). Diagnostic efficiency and hierarchical functioning of the DSM-IV borderline personality disorder criteria. *Journal of Nervous and Mental Disease, 187(3),* 167-173.

31. Widiger, T. A., Sanderson, C., & Warner, L. (1986). The MMPI, prototypal typology, and borderline personality disorder. *Journal of Personality Assessment, 51(2),* 228-242.

32. Clarkin, J. F., Widiger, T. A., Frances, A., Hurt, S. W., & Gilmore, M. (1983). Prototypic typology and the borderline personality disorder. *Journal of Abnormal Psychology, 93,* 263-275.

33. Snyder, S., Pitts, W. M., & Pokorny, A. D. (1986). Selected behavioral features of patients with borderline personality traits. *Suicide and Life Threatening Behavior, 16(1),* 28-39.

34. Stevens, A., Burkhardt, M., Hautzinger, M., Schwarz, J., Unckel, C. (2004) Borderline personality disorder: impaired visual perception and working memory. *Psychiatry Research, 125(3),* 257-67.

35. Hurt, S. W. & Clarkin, J. F. (1990). Borderline personality disorder: Prototypic typology and the development of treatment manuals. *Psychiatric Annals, 20(1)*: 13-18.

36. Blais, M.A., Hilsenroth, M.J., & Castlebury, F.D. (1997). Content validity of the DSM-IV borderline and narcissistic personality disorder criteria sets. *Comprehensive Psychiatry, 38(1),* 31-37.

37. Wilkinson-Ryan, R., & Westen, D. (2000). Identity disturbance in borderline personality disorder: An empirical investigation. *American Journal of Psychiatry, 157,* 528-541.

38. Fiqueroa, E.F., Silk, K.R. Huth, A. & Lohr, N.E. (1997). History of childhood sexual abuse and general psychopathology. *Comprehensive Psychiatry, 38 (1),* 23-30.

39. Kernberg, O. (1975). *Borderline conditions and pathological narcissism.* New York: Aronson.

40. Zanarini, M.C., Ruser, T.F., Frankenbur, F.R., Hennen, J., Gunderson, J.G. (2000). Risk factors associated with the dissociative experiences of borderline patients. *Journal of Nervous & Mental Diseases, 188(1),* 26-30.

41. Stein, K.F. (1996). Affect instability in adults with a borderline personality disorder. *Archives of Psychiatric Nursing, 10(1),* 32-40.

42. Leichsenring, F., Sachese, U. (2002). Emotions as wishes and beliefs. *Journal of Personality Assessment, 79(2),* 257-73.

43. Dougherty, D.M., Bjork, J.M., Huckabee, H.C., Moeller, F.G., & Swann, A.C. (1999). Laboratory measures of aggression and impulsivity in women with borderline personality disorder. *Psychiatry Research, 85(3),* 315-326.

44. Levine, D., Marziali, E. & Hood, J. (1997). Emotion processing in borderline personality disorders. *Journal of Nervous and Mental Disease, 185(4),* 240-246.

45. Paris, J., Zweig-Frank, H. (2001). A 27-year follow-up of patients with borderline personality disorder. *Comprehensive Psychiatry, 42(6),* 482-7.

46. Paris, J. (2002). Chronic suicidality among patients with borderline personality disorder. *Psychiatric Services, 53(6),* 738-42.

47. Kemperman, I., Russ, M.J., Shearin, E. (1997). Self-injurious behavior and mood regulation in borderline patients. *Journal of Personality Disorders, 11(2),* 146-157.

48. Welch, S.S., Linehan, M.M. (2002). High-risk situations associated with parasuicide and drug use in borderline personality disorder. *Journal of Personality Disorders, 16(6),* 561-9.

49. Barley, W. D., Thorward, S. R., Logue, M. A., McCready, K. F., Muller, J. P., Plakun, E. M., and Callahan, T. (1983). Characteristics of borderline personality disorder admissions to private psychiatric hospitals. *The Psychiatric Hospital, 17(4),* 195-199.

50. Leichsenring, F. (1999). Development and first results of the Borderline Personality Inventory: A self-report instrument for assessing borderline personality organization. *Journal of Personality Assessment, 73(1),* 45-63.

51. Zanarini, M.C., Vulganovic, A.A., Parachini, E.A., Boulanger, J.L., Frankenburg, F.R. Hennen, J. (2003). A screening measure for BPD: the McLean Screening Instrument for Borderline Personality Disorder (MSI-BPD). *Journal of Personality Disorders, 17(6),* 568-73.

52. Marziali, E., Muroe-Blum, H., & McCleary, L. (1999). The Objective Behavioral Index: A measure of assessing treatment response of patients with severe personality disorders. *Journal of Nervous & Mental Disorders, 187(5),* 290-295.

53. Morey, L.C. (1991). *Personality Assessment Inventory.* Odessa Fl: Psychological Assessment Resources, or San Antonio, TX: The Psychological Corporation.

54. Bell, P., Virginia, J., Pate, J.L., & Brown, R.C. (1997). Assessment of borderline personality disorder using the MMPI-2 and the Personality Assessment Inventory. *Assessment, 4(2),* 131-139.

55. Kurtz, J.E., Morey, L.C. (2001). Use of structured self-report assessment to diagnose borderline personality disorder during major depressive episodes. *Assessment, 8(3),* 291-300.

56. Zanarini, M. C., Gunderson, J. G., Frankenburg, F. R., & Chauncey, D. L. (1989). The revised diagnostic interview for borderlines: Discriminating BPD from other Axis II disorders. *Journal of Personality Disorders, 3(1),* 10-18.

57. Spitzer, R. L., Williams, J. B. W., & Gibbon, M. (1987). *Structured Clinical Interview for DSM-III-R.* New York: New York State Psychiatric Institute.

58. Fogelson, D. L., Nuechterlein, K. H., Asarnow, F.R., Subotnik, K.L., and Talovic, S.A. (1991). Interrater reliability of the Structured Clinical Interview for DSM-III-R, Axis II: Schizophrenia spectrum and affective spectrum disorders. *Psychiatry Research, 39(1),* 55-63.

59. Jacobsberg L., Perry S., Frances A. (1995) Diagnostic agreement between the SCID-II screening questionnaire and the Personality Disorder Examination. *J Pers Assess, 65(3):*428-33.

60. Zanarini, M.C., Vujanovic, A.A., Parachini, E.A., Boulanger, J.L., Frankenburg, F.R., Hennen, J. (2003). Zanarini Rating Scale for Borderline Personality Disorder (ZAN-BPD): A continuous measure of DSM-IV borderline psychopathology. *J Personal Disord 17(4):*1 p following 369.

61. Sansone, R.A., Wiederman, M.W., & Sansone, L.A. (1998). The Self-Harm Inventory (SHI): Development of a scale for identifying self-destructive behaviors and borderline personality disorder. *Journal of Clinical Psychology, 54(7),* 973-983.

62. Beck, A.T. (1991). *Beck Scale for Suicide Ideation (BSS).* San Antonio, TX: The Psychological Corporation.

63. Cull, J.G., & Gill, W.S. (1988). *Suicide Probability Scale.* Los Angeles, CA: Western Psychological Services.

64. Hathaway, S. R., Butcher, J.N., & McKinley, J. C. (1989). *Minnesota Multiphasic Personality Inventory-2.* Minneapolis, MN: University of Minnesota Press.

65. Zalewski, C. & Archer, R. P. (1991). Assessment of borderline personality disorder. *Journal of Nervous and Mental Diseases, 179(6),* 338-345.

66. Gartner, J. Hurt, S. W., Gartner, A. (1989). Psychological test signs of borderline personality disorder: A review of the empirical literature. *Journal of Personality Assessment, 53*(3), 423-441.

67. Graham, J. R. (1990). *MMPI-2: Assessing personality and psychopathology.* New York: Oxford University Press.

68. Kaufman, A. S. (1990). *Assessing adolescent and adult intelligence.* Boston: Allyn & Bacon, Inc.

69. Rapaport, D., Gill, M. M., & Schafer, F. (1945). *Diagnostic psychological testing.* (Vol. 1). Chicago: Year Book.

70. Exner. J.E. (1993). *The Rorschach: A comprehensive system; volume 1: Basic foundations.* Somerset, New Jersey: John Wiley and Sons.

71. Millon, T. (1987). *Millon clinical multi-axial inventory-II.* Minneapolis: National Computer Systems.

72. Kernberg, O. (1993). Suicidal behavior in borderline patients: Diagnosis and psychotherapeutic considerations. *American Journal of Psychotherapy, 47(2),* 245-254.

73. Brodsky, B.S., Malone, K.M., Ellis, S.P., Dulit, R.A., & Mann, J.J. (1997). Characteristics of borderline personality disorder associated with suicidal behavior. *American Journal of Psychiatry, 154 (12),* 1715-1719

74. Soloff, P.H., Lynch, K.G., Kelly, T.M., Malone, K.M., Mann, J.J. (2000) Characteristics of suicide attempts of patients with major depressive episode and borderline personality disorder: A comparative study. *American Journal of Psychiatry, 157(4),* 601-8.

75. Fine, M.A. & Sansone, R.A. (1990). Dilemmas in the management of suicidal behavior in individuals with borderline personality disorder. *American Journal of Psychotherapy, XLIV(2),* 160-169.

76. Borges, G., Walters, E.E., & Kessler, R.C. (2000). Associations of substance use, abuse, and dependence with subsequent suicidal behavior. *American Journal of Epidemiology, 151,* 781-789.

77. Kotsaftis, A. & Neale, J. M. (1993). Schizotypal personality disorder I: The clinical syndrome. *Clinical Psychology Review (Vol 13),* 451-472.

78. Perry, J. C., Herman, J. L., Van Der Kolk, B. A., & Hoke, L. A. (1990) . Psychotherapy and psychological trauma in borderline personality disorder. *Psychiatric Annals, 20(1),* 33-43.

79. Zanarini, M.C., Williams, A.A., Lewis, R.E., Reich, R.B., Vera, S.C., Marino, M.F., Levin, A., Yong, L., & Frankenburg, F.R. (1998). Reported pathological childhood experiences associated with the development of borderline personality disorder. *American Journal of Psychiatry, 154(8),* 1101-1106.

80. McLean, L.M., Gallop, R., (2003). Implications of childhood sexual abuse for adult borderline personality disorder and complex posttraumatic stress disorder. *American Journal of Psychiatry, 160(2),* 369-71.

81. Zanarini, M. C., Gunderson, J. G., Marino, M. F., Schwartz, E. O., & Frankenburg, F. R. (1989). Childhood experiences of borderline patients. *Comprehensive Psychiatry, 30(1),* 18-25.

82. Guzder, J., Paris, J., Selkowitz, P., & Feldman, R. (1999). Psychological risk factors for borderline pathology in school-age children. *Journal of the American Academy of Child & Adolescent Psychiatry, 38(2),* 206-212.

83. Loranger, A. W., Oldham, J. M., & Utlis, E. H. (1982). Familial transmission of DSM-III borderline personality disorder. *Archives of General Psychiatry, 39,* 795-799.

84. Loranger, A. W. & Tulis, E. H. (1985). Family history of alcoholism in borderline personality disorder. *Archives of General Psychiatry, 42,* 153-157.

85. Soloff, P. H. Millward, J. W. (1983). Psychiatric disorders in the families of borderline patients. *Archives of General Psychiatry, 40,* 37-44.

86. Pope, H. G., Jonas, J. M., & Hudson, J. I. et al. (1983). The validity of DSM-III personality disorder. *Archives of General Psychiatry, 40,* 23-30.

87. Zanarini, M. C. Genderson, J. F., & Marinio, J. F. et al. (Eds.) (1990). Psychiatric disorders in the families of borderline outpatients. *Family Environment and Borderline Personality Disorder.* Washington, D.C.: American Psychiatric Press.

88. Dubo, E.D., Zanarini, M.C., Lewis, R.E., & Williams, A.A. (1997). Childhood antecedents of self-destructiveness in borderline personality disorder. *Canadian Journal of Psychiatry, 42(1),* 63-69.

89. Kernberg, O. F., Selzer, M. A., Koenigsberg, H. W., Carr, A. C., Appelbaum, A. H. (1989). *Psychodynamic psychotherapy of borderline patients.* New York: Basic Books.

90. Sullivan, H.S. (1953). *The interpersonal theory of psychiatry.* New York: Norton.

91. Pollack, W.S. (1986). Borderline personality disorder: Definition, diagnosis, assessment and treatment considerations. *Innovations in clinical practice, 5,* 103-135.

92. Bryer, J. B., Nelson, B. A., Miller, F. B., & Krol, P. A. (1987). Childhood sexual and physical abuse as factors in adult psychiatric illness. *American Journal of Psychiatry, 144,* 1426-1430.

93. Piper, W.E., Rosie, J.S., Azim, H.F.A., & Joyce, A.S. (1993). A randomized trial of psychiatric day treatment for patients with affective and personality disorders. *Hospital Community Psychiatry, 44,* 757-763.

94. Clarkin, J.F., Foelsch, P.A., Levy, K.N., Hull, J.W., Delaney, J.C., Kernberg, O.F. (2001). The development of a psychodynamic treatment for patients with borderline personality disorder: A preliminary study of behavioral change. *Journal of Personality Disorders, 15(6),* 487-95.

95. Higgit, A. and Fonagy, P. (1992). Psychotherapy in borderline and narcissistic personality disorder. *British Journal of Psychiatry, 161,* 23-43.

96. Pazzagli, A., Monti, M.R. (2000). Dysphoria and aloneness in borderline personalitty disorder. *Psychopathology, 33(4),* 220-6.

97. Stern, M.I., Herron, W.G., Primavera, L.H., & Kakuma, T. (1997). Interpersonal perceptions of depressed and borderline inpatients. *Journal of Clinical Psychology, 53(1),* 41-49.

98. Bateman, A., & Fonagy, P. (1999). Effectiveness of partial hospitalizaion in the treatment of borderline personality disorder: A randomized controlled trial. *American Journal of Psychiatry, 156(10),* 1563-1569.

99. Bateman, A., Fonagy, P. (2001). Treatment of borderline personality disorder with psychoanalytically oriented partial hospitalization: An 18-month follow-up. *American Journal of Psychiatry, 158(1),* 36-42.

100. Bateman, A., Fonagy, P. (2003). Health service utilization costs for borderline personality disorder patients treated with psychoanalytically oriented partial hospitalization versus general psychiatric care. *American Journal of Psychiatry, 160(1),* 169-71.

101. Stevenson, J. & Meares, R. (1992). An outcome study of psychotherapy for patients with borderline personality disorder. *American Journal of Psychiatry, 149(3),* 358-362.

102. Waldinger R. J., Gunderson, J. F. (1984). Completed psychotherapies with borderline patients. *American Journal of Psychotherapy, 38(1),* 90-201.

103. Anchin, J. C. and Kiesler, D. J. (1982). *The handbook of interpersonal psychotherapy.* Elmsford, NY: Pergamon Press.

104. Coley, C. H. (1956). *Human nature and the social order.* Glencoe, IL: Free Press

105. Benjamin, L. S. (1974). Structural analysis of social behavior. *Psychological Review, 81,* 392-425.

106. Benjamin, L.S. (1993). *Interpersonal diagnosis and treatment of personality disorders.* New York, N.Y.: Guilford Press.

107. McKay, D., Gavigan, C.A., Kulchycky, S. (2004). Social skills and sex-role functioning in borderline personality disorder: relationship to self-mutilating behavior. *Cognitive Behavior Therapy, 33(1),* 27-35.

108. Shea et al. (1990). National institute of mental health multicentre trial of treatment for affective disorders. *American Journal of Psychiatry, 147,* 711-718.

109. Beck, A. T. & Arthur Freeman & Associates (1990). *Cognitive therapy of personality disorders.* New York: Guilford publications.

110. Butler, A.C., Brown, G.K., Beck, A.T., Grisham, J.R. (2002). Assessment of dysfunctional beliefs in borderline personality disorder. *Behaviour Research & Therapy, 40(10),* 1231-40.

111. Linehan, M. M. (1987). Dialectical behavior therapy for borderline personality disorder: Theory and methods. *Bulletin of the Menninger Clinic, 51,* 261-276.

112. Linehan, M.M. & Kehrer, C.A. (1993). Borderline personality Disorder. In D.H. Barlwo (Ed.), *Clinical Handbook of Psychological Disorders (2nd ed.).* New York: Guilford Press, 396-441

113. Heard, H.L. & Linehan, M.M. (1994). Dialectical behavior therapy: An integrative approach to the treatment of borderline personality disorder. *Journal of Psychotherapy Integration, 4(1),* 55-82.

114. Linehan, M.M. & Schmidt, H. (1995). The dialectics of effective treatment of borderline personality disorder. In W.O. O'Donohue & L. Krasner (Eds.), *Theories in behavior therapy.* Washington, D.C. American Psychological Association, 553-584.

115. McMain, S., Korman, L.M., Dimeff, L. (2001). Dialectical behavior therapy and the treatment of emotion dysregulation. *Journal of Clinical Psychology, 57(2),* 183-96.

116. Woodberry, K.A., Miller, A.L., Glinski, J., Indik, J., Mitchell, A.G. (2002). Family therapy and dialectical behavior therapy with adolescents: Part II: A theoretical review. *American Journal of Psychiatry, 56(4),* 585-602.

117. Lewis, M. & Haviland, J. M. (Eds.) (1993). *Handbook of emotions.* New York: Guilford Press.

118. Linehan, M.M. (1993). *Cognitive-behavioral treatment of borderline personality disorder.* New York: Guilford Press.

119. Kastenbaum, J. F. (Eds.) (1969). Death and bereavement in later life. *Death and bereavement.* Springfield, IL: Charles C. Thomas.

120. Linehan, M.M., Armstrong, H.E., Suearez, A., Allmon, D., & Heard, H.L. (1991). Cognitive-behavioral treatment of chronically parasuicidal borderline patients. *Archives of General Psychiatry, 48,* 1060-1064.

121. Linehan, M.M, Tutek, K., & Heard, H.L. (1992). Interpersonal and social treatment outcomes for borderline personality disorder. *Poster presented at the annual meeting of the Association of the Advancement of Behavior Therapy,* Boston, MA.

122. Linehan, M.M., Schmidt, H. III., Dimeff, L.A., Craft, J.C., Kanter, J., Comtois, K.A. (1999). Dialectical behavior therapy for patients with borderline personality disorder and drug-dependence. *American Journal on Addictions, 8(4),* 279-92.

123. Verheul, R., Van Den Bosch, L.M., Koeter, M.W., De Ridder, M.A., Stijen, T., Van Den Brink, W. (2003). Dialectical behavior therapy for women with borderline personality disorder: 12-month, randomised clinical trail in The Netherlands. *British Journal of Psychiatry, 182,* 135-40.

124. Van Den Bosch, L.M., Verheul, R., Schippers, G.M., Van Den Brink, W. (2002). Dialectical behavior therapy of borderline patients with and without substance use problems: Implementation and long-term effects. *Addictive Behaviors, 27(6),* 911-23.

125. Linehan, M.M., Heard, H.L. & Armstrong, H.E. (1992). Naturalistic follow-up of a behavioral treatment for chronically parasuicidal borderline patients. *Unpublished manuscript,* University of Washington, Seattle, WA.

126. Linehan, M.M., Tutek, D.A., Heard, H.L., & Armstrong, H.E. (1994). Interpersonal outcome of cognitive behavioral treatment for chronically suicidal borderline patients. *The American Journal of Psychiatry, 151(12),* 1771-1776.

127. Simpson, E.G., Yen, S., Costello, E., Rosen, K., Begin, A., Pistorello, J., Pearlstein, T. (2004). Combined dialectical behavior therapy and fluoxetine in the treatment of borderline personality disorder. *Journal of Clinical Psychiatry, 65(3),* 379-85.

128. Soler, J., Pascual, J.C., Campins, J., Barrachina, J., Puigdemont, D., Alvarez, E., Perez, V. (2005). Double-blind, placebo-controlled study of dialectical behavior therapy plus olanzapine for borderline personality disorder. *American Journal of Psychiatry, 162(6),* 1221-4.

129. Scheel, K.R. (2000). The emperical basis of dialectical behavior therapy: Summary, critique, and implications. *Clinical Psychology: Science and Practice, 7,* 68-86.

130. Wildgoose, A., Clarke, S., Waller, G. (2001). Treating personality fragmentation and dissociation in borderline personality disorder: A pilot study of the impact of cognitive analytic therapy. *British Journal of Medical Psychology, 74(Pt 1),* 47-55.

131. Ryle, A. (1997). The structure and development of borderline personality disorder: A proposed model. *British Journal of Psychiatry, 170,* 82-87.

132. Ryle, A., Leighton, T., & Pollock, P. (1997). *Cognitive analytic therapy and borderline personality disorder: The model and the method.* Chichister, England UK: John Wiley & Sons, Inc.

133. Ryle, A. (2000). Effectiveness of time-limited cognitive analytic therapy of borderline personaltiy disorder: Factors associated with outcome. *British Journal of Medical Psychology, 73(pt2),* 197-210.

134. Ryle, A. (1997). The structure and development of borderline personality disorder: A proposed model. *British Journal of Psychiatry, 170,* 82-87.

135. Parry, G. (1998). The accuracy of reformulation in cognitive analytic therapy: A validation study. *Psychotherapy Research, 8(1),* 84-103.

136. Ryle, A., Golynkina, K. (2000). Effectiveness of time-limited cognitive analytic therapy of borderline personality disorder: Factors associated with outcome. *British Journal of Medical Psychology, 73(Pt 2),* 197-210.

137. Marlett, G. A. & Gordon, J. R. (1985). *Relapse prevention.* New York: Guilford Press.

138. Waldinger, R.J. (1986). *Fundamentals of psychiatry.* Washington, D.C.: American Psychiatric Association.

139. Clarkin, J. F., Koenigsberg, H., Yeomans, F. et al. (1992). *Psychodynamic psychotherapy of the borderline patient in borderline personality disorder,* Ed's. Clarkin, J.F., Marziali, E., & Munroe-Blum, H. New York: Guilford Press.

140. McIntyre, S.M., & Scwartz, R.C. (1998). Therapists' differential countertransference reactions toward clients with major depression or borderline personality disorder. *Journal of Clinical Psychology, 54(7),* 923-931.

141. Yalom, I. D. (1985). *The theory and practice of group psychotherapy.* New York: Basic Books.

142. Clarkin, J. F., Marziali, E., & Munroe-Blum, H. (1991). Group and family treatments for borderline personality disorder. *Hospital and Community Psychiatry, 42(10),* 1038-1043.

143. Munroe-Blum, H., & Marziali, E. (1988). Time-limited group treatment of borderline personality disorder. *Can J Psychiatry, 33(5)*:364-9

144. Linehan, M. M. (1987b). Dialectical behavior therapy: A cognitive behavioral approach to parasuicide. *Journal of Personality Disorders, 1,* 328-333.

145. Nehls, N. (1991). Borderline personality disorder and group therapy. *Archives of Psychiatric Nursing, 3,* 137-146.

146. Bongar, B. (2002). *The suicidal patient: Clinical and legal standards of care (2nd Ed.).* Washington, DC: American Psychological Association.

147. Miller, L.J. (1989). Inpatient management of borderline personality disorder: A review and update. *Journal of Personality Disorders, 3(2),* 122-134.

148. Koenigsberg, H. (1984). Indications for hospitalization in the treatment of borderline patients. *Psychiatric Quarterly, 56,* 247-258.

149. Kernberg, O. F. (Eds.) (1982). Supportive psychotherapy with borderline conditions. *Critical Problems in Psychiatry.* Philadelphia: Lippincott.

150. Adler, G. (1985). *Borderline psychopathology and its treatment.* New York: Aronson.

151. White, T.W. (2003). Legal issues and suicide risk management. *The National Psychologist, 12(2),* 12.

152. Soloff, P. H.. & Millward, J. W. (1983). Developmental histories of borderline patients. *Comprehensive Psychiatry, 24,* 547-588.

153. Korzekwa, M., Links, P., and Steiner, M. (1993). Biological markers in borderline personality disorder: New perspectives. *American Journal of Psychiatry, 38(Suppl. 1),* S11-15.

154. De la Funete, J.M., Bobes, J., Vizuete, C., Mendlewicz, J. (2001). Sleep-EEG in borderline patients without concomitant major depression: A comparison with major depressives and normal control subjects. *Psychiatry Research, 105(1-2),* 87-95.

155. Coccaro, E. F. & Kavoussi, R. J. (1991). Biological and pharmacological aspects of borderline personality disorder. *Hospital and Community Psychiatry, 42(10),* 1029-1034.

156. Hirschfeld, R.M., (1997). Pharmacotherapy of borderline personality disorder. *Journal of Clinical Psychiatry, 58(suppl 14),* 48-52.

157. Coccaro, E.F. (1998). Clinical outcome of psychopharmacologic treatment of borderline and schizotypal personality disordered subjects. *Journal of Clinical Psychiatry, 59(suppl 1),* 30-35.

158. Steinberg, B.J., Trestman, R., Mitropoulou, V., Serby, M., Silverman, J., Coccaro, E., Weston, S., de Vegvar, M., & Siever, L.J. (1997). Depressive response to physostigmine challenge in borderline personality disorder patients. *Neuropsychopharmacology, 17(4),* 264-273.

159. Skodol, A.E., Siever, L.J., Livesley, W.J., Gunderson, J.G., Pfohl, B., Widiger, T.A. (2002). The borderline diagnosis II: biology, genetics and clinical course. *Biological Psychiatry, 51(12),* 951-63.

160. Judd, P. H., & Ruff, R. M. (1993). Neuropsychological dysfunction in borderline personality disorder. *Journal of Personality Disorders, 7(4),* 275-284.

161. Brown, G.L., Ebert, J.H., Goyer, P.F., Jimerson, D.C., Klein, W.J., Bunney, W.E. & Goodwin, F.K. (1982). Aggression, suicide & serotonin: Relationships to CSF amine metabilites. *American Journal of Psychiatry, 139(6)*, 741-746.

162. Verkes, R. J., Van der Mast, R.C., Kerkhof, A.J., Fekkes, D., Hengeveld, M.W., Tuyl, J.P., & Van Kempen, G. M. (1998). Platelet serotonin, monoamine oxidase activity, and [3H] paroxetine binding related to impulsive suicide attempts and borderline personality disorder. *Biological Psychiatry, 43(10)*, 740-746.

163. Choatai, J., Kullgren, G., & Asberg, M. (1998). CSF monoamine metabolites in relation to the diagnostic interview for borderline patients (DIB). *Neuropsychobiology, 38(4)*, 207.212.

164. Goodman, M., New, A. (2000). Impulsive appression in borderline personality disorder. *Current Psychiatry Reports, 2(1)*, 56-61.

165. Bronisch, T., Brunner, J., Bondy, B., et al. (2005). A multicenter study about neurobiology of suicidal behavior: Design, development, and preliminary results. *Arch Suicide Res 9(1)*: 19-26.

166. Rinne, T., Westenberg, H.G., den Boer, J.A., van den Brink, W. (2000). Serotonergic blunting to meta-chlorophenylpiperazine (m-CPP) highly correlates with sustained childhood abuse in impulsive and autoaggressive female borderline patients. *Biological Psychiatry, 47(6)*, 548-56.

167. Hansenne, M., Pitchot, W., Pinto, E., Reggers, J., Scantamburlo, G., Fuchs, S., Pirard, S., Ansseau, M. (2002). 5-HT1A dysfunction in borderline personality disorder. *Psychological Medicine, 32(5)*, 935-41.

168. De la Fuente, J.M., Tugendhaft, P., & Mavroudakis, N. (1998). Electroencephalographic abnormalities in borderline personality disorder. *Psychiatry Research, 77(2)*, 131-138.

169. Tebartz van Elst, L., Hesslinger, B., Thiel, T., Geiger, E., Haegele, K., Lemieux, L., Lieb, K., Bohus, M., Henning, J., Ebert, D. (2003). Frontolimbic brain abnormalities in patients with borderline personality disorder: A volumetric magnetic resonance imaging study. *Biological Psychiatry, 54(2)*, 163-71.

170. Bohus, M., Schmahl, C., Lieb, K. (2004). New developments in the neurobiology of borderline personality disorder. *Current Psychiatry Reports, 6(1)*, 43-50.

171. Donegan, N.H., Sanislow, C.A., Blumberg, H.P., Fulbright, R.K., Lacadie, C., Skudlarski, P., Gore, J.C., Olson, I.R., McGlashan, T.H., Wexler, B.E. (2003). Amygdala hyperactivity in borderline personality disorder: Implications for emotional dysregulation. *Biological Psychiatry, 54(11)*, 1284-93.

172. Herpertz, S.C., Kunert, H.J., Schwenger, U.B., Sass, H. (1999). Affective responsiveness in borderline personality disorder: A psychophysiological approach. *American Journal of Psychiatry, 156(10)*, 1550.

173. Meares, R., Melkonian, D., Gordon, E., Williams, L. (2005). Distinct pattern of P3a event-related potential in borderline personality disorder. *Neuroreport; 16(3)*, 289-93.

174. Sprock, J., Rader, T.J., Kendall, J.P., Yoder, C.Y. (2000). Neuropsychological functioning in patients with borderline personality disorder. *Journal of Clinical Psychology, 56(12)*, 1587-600.

175. Kunert, H.J., Dryecke, H.W., Sass, H., Herpertz, S.C. (2003). Frontal lobe dysfunctions in borderline personality disorder? Heuropsychological findings. *Journal of Personality Disorders, 17(6)*, 497-509.

176. Soloff, P.H. (1994). Is there any drug treatment of choice for the borderline patient? *Acta Psychiatric Scandinavia, 89(Suppl. 379)*, 50-55.

177. Silva, H., Jerez, S., Paredes, A., Salvo, J., Reneria, P., Ramirez, A., & Montes, C. (1997). Fluoxetine in the treatment of borderline personality disorder. *Actas Luso-Espanolas de Neurologia, Psiquiatria Y Ciencias Afines, 25(6)*, 391-395.

178. Raj, Y.P. (2004). Psychopharmacology of borderline personality disorder. *Current Psychiatry Reports,* 6(3), 225-31.

179. Ryden, G., Vinnars, B. (2002). Pharmacological treatment of borderline personality disorders: Several options for symptom reduction but nothing for the disorder per se. *Lakartidningen, 99(50)*, 5088-94.

180. Oldham, J.M., Bender, D.S., Skodol, A.E., Dyck, I.R., Sanislow, C.A., Yen, S., Grilo, C.M., Shea, M.T., Zanarini, M.C., Gunderson, E.J., McGlashan, T.H. (2004) Testing an APA practice guideline: Symptom-targeted medication utilization for patients with borderline personality disorder. *Journal of Psychiatry Practice, 10(3)*, 156-61.

181. Frankenburg, F.R., Zanarini, M.C. (2002). Divalproex sodium treatment of women with borderline personality disorder and bipolar II disorder: A double-blind placebo-controlled pilot study. *Journal of Clinical Psychologyy,63(5)*, 442-6.

182. Hollander, E., Allen, A., Lopez, R.P., Bienstock, C.A., Grossman, R., Siever, L.J., Merkatz, L., Stein, D.J. (2001). A preliminary double-blind, placebo-controlled trail of divalproex sodium in borderline personality disorder. *Journal of Clinical Psychology, 62(3),* 199-203.

183. Rinne, T. van den Brink, W., Wouters, L., van Dyck, R. (2002). SSRI treatment of borderline personality disorder: A randomized, placebo-controlled clinical trail for female patients with borderline personality disorder. *American Journal of Psychiatry, 159(12),* 2048-54.

184. Zanarini, M.C., Frankenburg, F.R. (2001). Olanzapine treatment of female borderline personality disorder patients: A double-blind, placebo-controlled pilot study. *Journal of Clinical Psychiatry, 62(11),* 849-54.

185. Bogenschutz, M.P., George Nurnberg, H. (2004). Olanzapine versus placebo in the treatment of borderline personality disorder. *Journal of Clinical Psychiatry, 65(1),* 104-9

186. Zanarini, M.C., Frankenburg, F.R., Parachini, E.A. A preliminary, randomized trial of fluoxetine, olanzapine, and the olanzapine-fluoxetine combination in women with borderline personality disorder. *J Clin Psychiatry;* 2004 Jul;65(7):903-7

187. Nickel, M.K., Nickel, C., Mitterlehner, F.O., Tritt, K., Lahmann, C., Leiberich, P.K., Rother, W.K., Loew, T.H. (2004). Topiramate treatment of aggression in female borderline personality disorder patients: A double-blind, placebo-controlled study. *Journal of Clinical Psychiatry, 65(11),* 1515-9.

188. Zanarini, M.C., Frankenburg, F.R. (2003). Omega-3 fatty acid treatment of women with borderline personality disorder: A double-blind, placebo-controlled pilot study. *American Journal of Psychiatry, 160(1),* 167-9.

189. Rinne, T., de Kloet, E.R., Wouters, L., Goekoop, J.G., de Rijk, R.H., van den Brink, W. (2003). Fluvoxamine reduces responsiveness of HPA axis in adult female BPD patients with a history of sustained childhood abuse. *Neuropsychopharmacology, 28(1),* 126-32.

190. Chengappa, K.N.R., Ebeling, T., Kang, J.S., Levine, J., & Parepally, H. (1999). Clozapine reduces severe self-mutilation and aggression in psychotic patients with borderline personality disorder. *Journal of Clinical Psychiatry, 60(7),* 477-484.

191. Bendetti, F., Sforzini, L., Colombo, C., Marrei, C., & Smeraldi, E. (1998). Low-dose clozapine in acute and continuation treatment of severe borderline personality disorder. *Journal of Clinical Psychiatry, 59(3),* 103-107.

192. Rocca, P., Marchiaro, L., Cocuzza, E., Bogetto, F. (2002). Treatment of borderline personality disorder with risperidone. *Journal of Clinical Psychiatry, 63(3),* 241-4.

193. Hollander, E., Swann, A.C., Coccaro, E.F., Jiang, P., Smith, T.B. (2005). Impact of trait impulsivity and state aggression on divalproex versus placebo response in borderline personality disorder. *American Journal of Psychiatry, 162(3),* 621-4.

194. Pinto, O.C., Akiskal, H.S. (1998). Lamotrigine as a promising approach to borderline personality: an open case series without concurrent DSM-IV major mood disorder. *Journal of Affective Disorders, 51(3),* 333-43.

195. Bohus, M.J., Landwehrmeyer, G.B., Stiglmayr, C.E., Limberger, M.F., Bohme, R., & Schmahl, C.G. (1999). Naltrexone in the treatment of dissociative symptoms in patients with borderline personality disorder: An open-label trial. *Journal of Clinical Psychiatry, 60(9),* 598-603.

196. Philipsen, A., Richter, H., Schmahl, C., Peters, J., Rusch, N., Bohus, M., Lieb, K. (2004). Clonidine in acute aversive inner tension and self-injurious behavior in female patients with borderline personality disorder. *Journal of Clinical Psychiatry, 65(10),* 1414-9.

# Index

## S

Schizophrenia  14, 15, 57, 58

Schizophrenic  1, 15

Schizotypal personality disorder (SPD)  9, 17

Self-destructive behaviors  4, 7, 8, 10, 12,
    13, 17, 19, 23, 27, 50  *See also* Suicide

Self-harm  8, 12, 13, 27, 28, 31,
    38  *See also* Self-mutilation

Self-image  6, 7, 17, 47

Self-mutilation  6, 8, 9, 10, 19, 30, 36,
    41, 52, 58  *See also* Self-harm

Self-report  15

Self-report instruments  10, 12–13
    Borderline Personality Inventory  12
    McLean Screening Instrument
        for Borderline Personality
        Disorder (MSI-BPD)  12
    Objective Behavioral Index  12
    Personality Assessment
        Inventory (PAI)  12

Sertraline  62

Sexual
    Abuse  4, 7, 10, 19, 40
    Promiscuity  1, 6, 8, 9, 39, 40

Side effects  *See* Medication: Side effects

SSNRIs (Selective serotonin norepinephrine
    reuptake inhibitors)  61, 62  *See*
    *also* individual medications

SSRIs (Selective serotonin reuptake inhibitors)
    44, 61, 62  *See also* individual medications

Structured Clinical Interview for DSM-III-
    R Personality Disorders (SCID-II)  13

Subgroups of BPD  9

Substance abuse  3, 4, 6, 8, 10, 17, 19, 38, 40

Suicide  24, 28, 40, 43
    Assessment  6, 8, 9, 10, 13, 16
    Contracts  23, 53–54
    Managing suicide risk  52–55
    Parasuicidal behaviors  43, 52, 58
    Treatment
        Key treatment issues  55
        Psychotherapy  54

Suicide/self-harm assessment instruments  13
    Beck Scale for Suicide Ideation  13
    Self-Harm Inventory (SHI)  13
    Suicide Probability Scale (SPS)  13

Symptoms  1, 2, 3
    and assessment  6, 7, 9, 10, 14, 17
    and pharmacotherapy  58, 60, 61, 62–63
    and psychotherapy  33, 35, 43, 52, 53, 54

## T

Thioridazine  62

Topiramate  60, 63

Trauma  3
    and assessment  10, 17
    and pharmacotherapy  58
    and psychotherapy  19, 20,
        23, 26, 27, 28, 30, 40
    Post-traumatic stress disorder
        (PTSD)  9, 17

Treatment  *See* Pharmacological;
    Psychotherapy
    Efficacy
        of medications  60–64
        of psychotherapy  24, 28, 33, 44, 52
    Examples  25, 29, 32, 37, 44, 49

## V

Valproic acid  *See* Divalproex sodium

Venlafaxine  62

## W

Wechsler Adult Intelligence Scale-
    Revised (WAIS-R)  13, 14

## Z

Zanarini Rating Scale for Borderline
    Personality Disorder (ZAN-BPD)  13

Ziprasidone  62

# We Want Your Opinion!

*Comments about* **Borderline Personality Disorder**:

_____

_____

_____

_____

_____

*Other titles you would like Compact Clinicals to offer:*

_____

_____

_____

_____

*To be placed on our mailing list, please provide the following:*

Name: _____

Address: _____

_____

_____

E-mail: _____

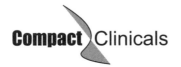

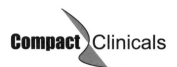

# Order in 3 easy steps:

## ▶ 1   Provide complete billing and shipping information

Name _____    Company _____

Profession _____    Dept./Mail Stop _____

Street Address/P.O. Box _____

City/State/Zip _____

Telephone _____    ☐ Ship to Residence   ☐ Ship to Business

## ▶ 2   Choose Titles

*For Clinicians:*

| | Qty. | Unit Price | Total |
|---|---|---|---|
| **Attention Deficit Hyperactivity Disorder**<br>*The latest assessment and treatment strategies* | | $16.95 | |
| **Bipolar Disorder**<br>*The latest assessment and treatment strategies* | | $16.95 | |
| **Borderline Personality Disorder**<br>*The latest assessment and treatment strategies* | | $16.95 | |
| **Conduct Disorders**<br>*The latest assessment and treatment strategies* | | $16.95 | |
| **Depression in Adults**<br>*The latest assessment and treatment strategies* | | $16.95 | |
| **Obsessive Compulsive Disorder**<br>*The latest assessment and treatment strategies* | | $16.95 | |
| **Post-Traumatic and Acute Stress Disorders**<br>*The latest assessment and treatment strategies* | | $16.95 | |

*For Physicians:*

| | | Unit Price | Total |
|---|---|---|---|
| **Bipolar Disorder: Treatment and Management** | | $18.95 | |

*Continuing Education credits available for mental health professionals. Call 1-800-408-8830 for details.*

| | |
|---|---|
| **Subtotal** | |
| **Tax** (Add 7.975% in MO) | |
| **Shipping** ($3.75 first book/ $1.00 per additional book) | |
| **TOTAL** | |

## ▶ 3   Choose Payment Method

Please charge my:   ☐ Visa   ☐ MasterCard   ☐ Discover   ☐ American Express    ☐ Check Enclosed

Account # __ __ __ __ — __ __ __ __ — __ __ __ __ — __ __ __ __    Exp. Date __ __ / __ __

Name on Card _____   Cardholder Signature _____

**Postal Orders:** Compact Clinicals, 7205 NW Waukomis Dr., Suite A, Kansas City, MO 64151

**Telephone Orders:** Toll Free 1-800-408-8830      **Fax Orders:** 1(816)587-7198

# We Want Your Opinion!

*Comments about* **Borderline Personality Disorder**:

_____

_____

_____

_____

_____

*Other titles you would like Compact Clinicals to offer:*

_____

_____

_____

_____

*To be placed on our mailing list, please provide the following:*

Name: _____

Address: _____

_____

_____

E-mail: _____

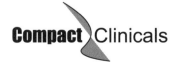

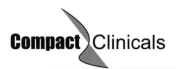

# Order in 3 easy steps:

## ▶ 1   Provide complete billing and shipping information

Name _____    Company _____

Profession _____    Dept./Mail Stop _____

Street Address/P.O. Box _____

City/State/Zip _____

Telephone _____    ☐ Ship to Residence    ☐ Ship to Business

## ▶ 2   Choose Titles

| For Clinicians: | Qty. | Unit Price | Total |
|---|---|---|---|
| **Attention Deficit Hyperactivity Disorder** <br> *The latest assessment and treatment strategies* | | $16.95 | |
| **Bipolar Disorder** <br> *The latest assessment and treatment strategies* | | $16.95 | |
| **Borderline Personality Disorder** <br> *The latest assessment and treatment strategies* | | $16.95 | |
| **Conduct Disorders** <br> *The latest assessment and treatment strategies* | | $16.95 | |
| **Depression in Adults** <br> *The latest assessment and treatment strategies* | | $16.95 | |
| **Obsessive Compulsive Disorder** <br> *The latest assessment and treatment strategies* | | $16.95 | |
| **Post-Traumatic and Acute Stress Disorders** <br> *The latest assessment and treatment strategies* | | $16.95 | |

*For Physicians:*

| | Qty. | Unit Price | Total |
|---|---|---|---|
| **Bipolar Disorder: Treatment and Management** | | $18.95 | |

| | |
|---|---|
| **Subtotal** | |
| **Tax** (Add 7.975% in MO) | |
| **Shipping** ($3.75 first book/ $1.00 per additional book) | |
| **TOTAL** | |

*Continuing Education credits available for mental health professionals. Call 1-800-408-8830 for details.*

## ▶ 3   Choose Payment Method

Please charge my:   ☐ Visa   ☐ MasterCard   ☐ Discover   ☐ American Express    ☐ Check Enclosed

Account # __ __ __ __ — __ __ __ __ — __ __ __ __ — __ __ __ __    Exp. Date __ __ / __ __

Name on Card _____    Cardholder Signature _____

**Postal Orders:** Compact Clinicals, 7205 NW Waukomis Dr., Suite A, Kansas City, MO 64151

**Telephone Orders:** Toll Free 1-800-408-8830      **Fax Orders:** 1(816)587-7198